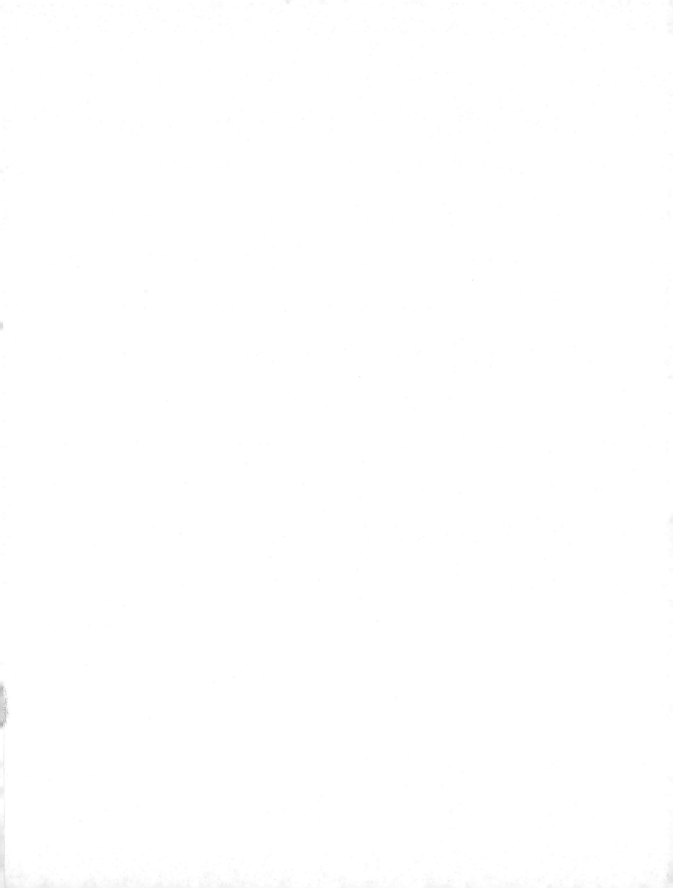

Principles of Teaching Yoga to Kids

A Complete guide on How to teach yoga to kids in a fun, creative and most effective way

NOBIEH KIANI FARD

BALBOA.PRESS

A DIVISION OF HAY HOUSE

Balboa Press books may be ordered through booksellers or by contacting:

Balboa Press
A Division of Hay House
1663 Liberty Drive
Bloomington, IN 47403
www.balboapress.com
844-682-1282

Print information available on the last page.

ISBN: 978-1-9822-5383-7 (sc)
ISBN: 978-1-9822-5384-4 (e)

Balboa Press rev. date: 09/18/2020

"Every Child is an Artist. The problem is how to remain as Artist once He grows up" Pablo Picasso

Contents

Author's Word

"In the Name of Love, Friendship
&
the beloved Inner Child of You All"
Namaste!

I am Nobieh Kianifard. I started teaching yoga to children between 5 to 12 years old in my home country Tehran, Iran in 1999. I am always thankful that the foundation of my educational career was based on working with children.

Spending time with children taught me how to be present in the moment, and be able to hold a diverse and pleasant class for them with more creativity and greater ideas in each session. Each class was a learning session for me. I got to know myself better along with children, through observing them, and with their help, I came up with creative ideas and plans. This made me discover more about them and their mysterious world in order to introduce yoga to them, as a gift in the best possible way.

During the years I taught yoga to kids, everything was becoming an inspiration for me and I was thinking and writing for hours, reflecting on how to bring a new idea into my yoga class. I got inspired from watching animations, observing nature and all the creatures, the way they move and their behavior to the inspiring stories, poetries, books, kids psychology articles and books on how to communicate better with kids, creative games and mostly just by observing kids playing and communicating among each other.

After working for some time with that first group of kids I started my journey of sharing yoga with, I wrote a story based on yoga asanas and named it: "Our Magical jungle of yoga". We performed it for their parents in the form of a play and since "The magical Jungle of yoga" became the main name for my yoga kids' classes.

Sharing all these ideas and witnessing their joy and excitement inspired me to expand my research then I provided children with more diverse, useful, and professional techniques every year.

I shared "The magical jungle of yoga" with children from different countries. Later, feeling that it was necessary to make that unique experience accessible to more children, I started to design a teacher training course to educate yoga teachers to specifically work with kids, and in 2006, I performed the first 35-hour yoga kids teacher training course for Iran Yoga Association. The course was held in Tehran and other cities, then I expanded the teaching worldwide also. Over the years, the length of the training course increased.

Nobieh yoga kids teacher training program is now 110 hours long, being held in Nobieh school of yoga registered with yoga alliance since 2014. (RCYS) (Restricted Children Yoga School).

The circle of" our Magical Jungle of yoga" is getting bigger every year. This magic is expanded in different countries by the prominent instructors, being graduated from these training sessions.

In this book I gathered a practical and complete training manual in a way for you to be able to use it and bring lots of joy into the kid you will be introducing these insights with…

It was such an honor and heart touching experience for me to witness all the joy, laughter, fun and emotional moments my adult trainees were going through by healing their own inner child in these training sessions.

I cannot reflect the amazing feelings we shared during these years in all the magical circles of yoga kids TTC, but In this training book, I shared all the useful information and ideas you can take into your own yoga sessions and witness the magic by yourself!

I hope a day comes when all of us live together, with harmony, peace and unity, in a magical jungle of love. I hope a day comes when we learn to accept each other, love each other unconditionally and give color and beauty to our world with our inner magic. I hope we also teach this to our children, to create a world as beautiful and colorful as **"Our Magical Jungle of yoga"**.

Preface

Kids are the original yogis. In many ways, they develop their own asana because of their natural flexibility. Bending backwards and forwards for instance, is much easier and fun for them to do. In this book you will learn how to create varied and fun classes for children of all ages.

Games will be explained in a simple way. You will experience each and every game and connect with your inner kid, then you'll be ready to introduce it in the world of children.

With your knowledge and creativity, you will be prepared to develop your own way of teaching yoga to children of different abilities and ages.

We go through this process together because we have all been kids before, we love kids, we work with kids and some of us have their own kids we want to share this magic with them.

Our purpose and goal through this process and teachings is to understand children's abilities and limits, to then design & create dynamic, entertaining, useful and amazing classes just for them.

Enjoy the journey. Free your mind, play like a kid, have fun, and laugh a lot!

How and for whom this book is written:

First, I want to thank you for choosing this training book and welcome you to the exciting world of yoga for kids.

My goal of writing this book was to give you a complete, practical guide to understand children's world, design fun and effective yoga sessions for kids, but also to know better your own inner child and enjoy experiencing life with yoga and **play as a child.**

This book **is written for** Yoga teachers or yoga practitioners who like to share yoga with their kids.

One thing I want to point out here is that this book is not illustrated but will guide you step by step into how to execute a game and take the ideas into designing your yoga session for kids.

Also, **in this book you won't learn** about how to teach yoga asanas in their traditional way and their exact teaching points and adjustments.

So, if you don't know the yoga asanas, you might get confused and you need to be a yoga teacher or a passionate and regular yoga practitioner to get more benefit from this book.

Also, if you come with any questions during your reading, you can always drop me an email and I'll be happy to assist you in your process.

I wish you a pleasant journey on reading and applying this book into your yoga sessions.

Nobieh
www.nobiehkiani.com
nobieh@nobiehkiani.com

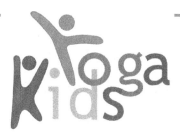

CHAPTER 1
Meaning of yoga, why yoga for kid and how?

The Meaning of Yoga:

Now that you are reading this book, you might be a yoga instructor, passionate about yoga, a parent who likes to share your yoga practice with your kids and thus have enough information about yoga. However, it is better to briefly discuss the "meaning of yoga", before getting into the subjects related to children yoga:

Yoga means unity. One of the goals of yoga is to bring harmony and integrity between mind, soul and body. Yoga is an ancient science which deals with having a healthy body and soul, calming the mind, composing thoughts and improving the quality of material and spiritual communications.

The exact time and the reason for the emergence of yoga is unknown, but around 3000 years ago, the basics of yoga were collected by an enlightened sage named Patanjali, who was one the greatest yogis. These basics were then compiled in a book named "Yogasutra" for the first time.

Patanjali presented yoga in eight main sections, which are briefly as follows:

Eight Limbs of Yoga:

The path of yoga leads us to acknowledge the spiritual aspects of our nature.

The following eight steps are practical guidelines on how to live a meaningful, purposeful life leading into a healthy body & mind also connecting to our soul purpose.

The eight Limbs of yoga to which Patanjali has pointed in the book "Yogasutra" are as follows:

1- Yama : Ethical rules and Morality
2- Nyama : Self-discipline and personal observances
3- Asana : Yoga postures
4- Pranayama : Managing the breath and the energy force within
5- Pratyahara : Withdrawal Of senses
6- Dharana : Concentration
7- Dhyana : Meditation
8- Samadhi : Union, Oneness

Yama:
1- Harmlessness and nonviolence (Ahimsa)
2- Truthfulness and honesty (Satya)
3- Non-Stealing, Righteousness (Asteya)
4- Virtue of managing senses and being free of greed (Brahmacharya)
5- Non Possessiveness, Not attaching to things (Aparigraha)

Niyama:
1- Cleanliness and observing personal health (Saucha)
2- Satisfaction and contentment (Santosh)
3- Self-cultivation (Tapas)
4- Self-seeking and studying spiritual books (Svadhyaya)
5- Surrendering to the supreme consciousness (Ishvarapranidhana)

Asana:

Asana relates to physical and bodily conditions. Body is like a sanctuary for the soul. We care for our bodies so that our souls rejoice!

Pranayama:

Prana is the energy of life and the meaning of Pranayama is controlling the energy of life. Pranayama are respiratory exercises of yoga that increase the lungs volume. Since during these exercises, the mind is completely focused on them, they calm the mind and increase its concentration. The deeper we breathe, the calmer our minds become.

Pratyahara:

The withdrawal of five senses. Observing our habits & taking a look at our attachments to our desires stopping us from our inner growths.

Dharna:

Concentration.

Slowing down the thinking process by concentrating our mind in a single object such as a specific point in our body, an image, a word or a mantra.

This stage is a preparation for meditation.

Dhyana:

Mediation begins in this stage; the mind is quieted and stillness happens.

A stage where the mind is free and released. The heart opens and the experience of being in the moment happens.

Samadhi:

Connection to the Divine; A state of ecstasy, pure joy and unity. It is like connecting to the whole universe.

The Necessity of Yoga Practice

Due to population growth and the rapid advancement of technology and urban life, human beings are becoming more and more oblivious of their bodies and souls and are drowning in the attractive and crowded appearance of modernity. The result is that they are confronted with a troubled and confused mind, a tired body and physical and mental contractions and knots. Although the effectiveness of yoga, physical, respiratory and mental exercises are very beneficial in other situations, in such an environment, the necessity to use them is certainly felt more.

The mind and the body are completely interconnected. You must have experienced that if we have the slightest pain in a part of our physical body, we will definitely suffer from mental restlessness and lack of concentration. Conversely, if we have the slightest disturbance in our thoughts, the body will show disease-like reactions.

There are currently a variety of sports that exist in the world that can help keep our body healthy. Also, various methods and books are published every day in different parts of the world to calm and control the various thoughts and skills of life. But the problem is that each of these methods deals with a single aspect of human existence and neglects others. Fortunately, it can be explicitly claimed that yoga exercises deal with physical, mental and spiritual aspects at the same time. A healthy body, a calm mind and a free spirit are the presents yoga exercises and teachings offer you.

How can yoga impact children's lives?

Being a child again: Let's go back to childhood together; Back to the time when excitement had a meaning, back to the time of innocence, when colors had meaning, the days when some of us still believed in the magical world of angels. Let's all see the world once again from a child's eyes and believe that we can change our lives with the power of love. Let's all experience being a kid again in order to connect to them from their perspective.

When we use the word "magical" for children, we explain that magic is real and it is energy that exists within us, for instance: love, kindness, friendship, courage, knowledge, peace and so on. With this magic we give kids wings to fly, but we also need to give them roots to ground themselves.

They need a secure and lovable environment to have wings to fly, and support to fix their roots in the ground.

WHAT THE CLASSES CAN PROVIDE FOR CHILDREN

Create an 'ideal' body: The tools given in this process will help achieve control, balance, power and stamina. Breathing exercises will increase the size of their lungs and create calm.

Increase sensory awareness: By becoming more in touch with their bodies, breath and creativity they will be able to perceive circumstances outside the classroom with more sensitivity.

Communication and creativity: Through use of group activities children learn to develop communication skills, trust of others and confidence in their own creativity.

Which Asanas? In choosing which asanas and games you provide for your classes your main concern will be age and ability level. What is suitable and fun for the younger children won't achieve the same results with the older children.

*Age groups are described later in the chapter related to "Practical info for instructors".

The use of yoga in School environments:

Yoga does not have to be taught in a studio or a gymnasium. It can be taught in a simple classroom or a small space. For example, you can do some of the exercises while sitting on a chair instead of sitting or lying on the ground. You can calm the children down by practicing breathing exercises for busier classes. This brings balance to their behavior.

Yoga held in schools, will not disrupt their education, it will only improve it.

The atmosphere of the class

When choosing a location for your yoga class, it is important to find somewhere that has enough space for the children to express themselves and provides a comfortable environment for them to jump around and make noise. If there are no mats, make sure they bring one, plus a blanket and towel. It allows kids to make their own space.

Having a cushion will make sitting more comfortable. Many of the games use music as well, so having a music system is necessary. Importantly, the floor must be clean.

You should keep the windows open during breathing exercises.

Why Yoga for Children?

Given all the benefits and positive effects that physical and mental yoga exercises can have on a person's life, it would be so great if we learn and use them since childhood. These days, children are in dire need of a more accurate knowledge of themselves and their bodies, need to become more acquainted with their thoughts and feelings, and better understand the real and healthy relation with those around them. It is obvious that such children will be more successful, happier and calmer adults, since childhood experiments have a direct impact on personality formation in adulthood. Children at a very young age are in a way yogis by nature. Just look at them while playing, and realize that they are naturally and unexpectedly doing some of the yoga postures, such as "Down-ward dog", "Child pose", "Bridge", etc. They also create their own movements. Since they are highly flexible, many back bends and reverse postures are very easy and fun to do for them.

In this book, you will learn how to design a diverse, joyful and creative class for children. The games are explained in a simple language and a dynamic, practical way. With a thorough study of the book, applying the ideas and using your own creativity, you can design a creative, fun but also educational program for kids.

Our only goal and focus in this book is "children with all their abilities and limitations".

Let us take a look at the benefits of yoga for children:

- Improves strength and flexibility
- Increases self-confidence, provides a positive self-image
- Increases emotional power
- Nurture creativity
- Helps to balance mind and body
- Teaches self-acceptance and self-love
- Increases sensory awareness and general body awareness
- Creates balance and harmony
- Improves awareness of self and others
- Develops discipline and self-control
- Helps to improve mental concentration
- Helps having a strong body as well as a stretched and flexible spinal cord
- Reinforces bodily systems: bones, nervous system, blood circulatory system, gastrointestinal system, respiratory system, hormones, and muscles, and increases the knowledge about the body anatomy
- Increases respiratory awareness and helps taking deeper breaths
- Encourage cooperation and teamwork
- Improves the understanding of anatomy
- Develops awareness of nature, animals and environment
- Helps to improve willpower
- Teaches how to keep calm and reduce anxiety
- Encourages kindness, generosity, and respect
- Teaches how to find peace from inside
- And pay attention to the point that:
  "Yoga is so joyful and fun!"

It should be noted that teaching yoga to children is completely different from teaching it to adults. High energy and excitement of children make them unable to sit still in silence for a long time. They refuse to listen to the deep mental and spiritual concepts and such exercises. Therefore, to convey yoga to children with the highest productivity, we should first enter their world and discover the language of communicating with them. This is very simple, since all of us have been a child some time. So, close your eyes for a moment and remember the time when enthusiasm and bewilderment were meaningful to you, the time of innocence, safety, confidence, fantasy and creativity.

Now let us go back to the sweet childhood; The time of a colorful world of imagination. The time when we still had faith in the mysterious world of angels, fairies, and magic. Let us once again watch the world from the pure eyes of a child, and believe that we can change the world around us with the magic of "love".

Let us once again experience "being a child" along with the children.

Welcome to the "Magical Jungle of Love" we call YOGA!

The Magical Jungle of yoga:

First of all, it is better if we briefly explain the word "Magic". This is a word that I, myself use in my classes very often. When we use "magic" for children, we must explain to them that magic is true. Magic exists inside all of us. In fact, our magic is our very inner powers such as love, kindness, friendship, courage, awareness, peace and…..

Later In the chapter of "Colors & their impacts", you will learn how we can make children understand their emotions more and more, by spreading different colors along with our specific magic, which are actually our inner energies.

…And the story of Our Magical jungle of yoga…

Our Magical jungle is a name I have chosen for my children yoga classes, and now I'm going to take you into a beautiful journey in this magical and creative world:

(Follow the story and when you encounter a yoga posture (Asana) take yourself and your kids into the posture then continue to play along with the story and enjoy the journey!)

Our Magical Jungle

Once upon a time, under the shiny blue sky, at a corner of this crowded city, there was a magical jungle…

In this magical jungle, we have a magical colorful sunflower (children are sitting round in a circle), each petal of which has one color and spreads a special magic in our jungle (each child in the circle says their color and magic).

Yellow petal: magic of hope….

Pink petal: magic of love and friendship….

Sky blue petal: magic of peace…

Orange petal: magic of creativity….

Green petal: magic of health….

Dark blue petal: magic of bravery and courage….

Red petal: magic of excitement…

Purple petal: magic of intuition…

Every morning, when our petals gather together with the rising of the shiny sun, say prayers and gather their energies, they are ready to spread their energy inside our magical jungle… gradually they begin "The Magical Flower Dance" (Sun salutation), later the wind starts blowing and spreading all those colorful petals through our magical Jungle….

First, they turn into enchanted trees that make all wishes come true (Vrikshasana), then they become warriors who fight with evil and darkness with their positive vibes and magic sparks; They are warriors of love (Virabhadrasana). Since our jungle is magical, trees can be upside down, stand on their foliage and observe everywhere and everything from down to the top in order to prevent any little devil from entering the jungle secretly! (Adho mukha svanasana).

Then they all turn into bridges for everyone who wants to pass under; a bridge that pours its specific magic inside them. (Urdhva Dhanurasana)

They then become bows to form a beautiful magical rainbow. (Dhanurasana)

They can turn into camels and spread patience(Ustrasana).

Or become cute kittens who always know how lovely they are…(Marjariasana)

Or dogs who are kind and loyal friends… (Urdhva Mukha svanasana)

They know, and tell everyone how good it is to sometimes see the world from another angle (Uttanasana), they can be birds flying (Crow pose), unbound and free, high in the sky in search of the Phoenix, become turtles who, slowly and continuously, go on their ways (Kurmasana), and then turn into colored beautiful butterflies who fly and spread their magic all around the jungle (Baddha Konasana).

On the birthday of the Lion jungle (Simhasana), they sit round in a circle and become candles; each, with their own color and light, makes a wish for our Lion (Sarvangasana). When the Lion comes and blows out the candles, they go off (Halasana) and come back to eat the cake together, Dandasana then (Paschimottanasana).

Then, they turn into small colorful fishes and, with their pure hearts, like the pure flowing water, they float in the ocean of life (Matsyasana), Going with the flow and letting the water take them into the next adventure...

Before sunset, children turn into archeries (Akarna Dhanurasana), and for the last time in a wonderful adventurous day, they spread their wishes into the Magical jungle. These arrows fill everyone who encounters them with their colorful magic!

The sun is slowly setting, and our petals which spread their energy throughout the day in our Magical Jungle are now lying on the ground (Shavasana).

...and one by one, relax all body parts. The right leg comes up and is released, the left leg comes up and is released, hips come up and is released, rib cage comes up and is released on the ground, neck turns right, left, middle and is released, they gather their faces as if their whole faces go to the tip of their noses, then they make a deep roar like a lion announcing the end of a good and lovely day in our magical forest, and make a circle again...

Now, all the petals are released, and from their hearts they spread their beautiful colors inside the circle of our Magical jungle!

Now, a world of energy and colorful lights has spread throughout their bodies, and fill them with magical energies of love, peace, kindness, courage, vitality, creativity, excitement and health.

While these colorful sparkles are surrounding them like a beautiful rainbow, they tightly embrace themselves and feel how loveable and beautiful they are; then they bend their knees, turn to their right side, allowing the loving mother earth to nurture them in her arms. After that, they sit up in the shape of a beautiful lotus flower (Padmasana), and while growing higher toward the sunlight, they take each other's hands, unite and pray:

Big as a giant

small as a peanut
we're all the same size
in our Magical Jungle of yoga

Nobieh Kiani fard

Wealthy as a king
poor as a mite
we are all worth the same
in our Magical Jungle of yoga
Black, red and purple
orange, yellow and white
we all look the same
in our Magical Jungle
So maybe the way
to make everything right
is for God to reach out
and turn every place like our Magical Jungle of yoga!
(lyrics inspired from Sel Silverstein poem)

Now they make a wish in their hearts and put it into the universe…

You can use the same story in your sessions and many other ideas and themes you will learn throughout this book and design your classes upon it.

In this book, I shared my experiences of teaching yoga to different groups of children during the years, Hoping to bring more awareness now in us as adults to educate our kids to become happier, healthier and more joyful, compassionate and caring human beings!

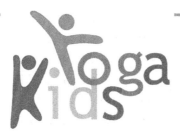

CHAPTER 2

Characteristics of a Successful kids Yoga Instructor

- It is good to know that you need a high level of energy to work with children. Being energetic is a characteristic of children, and a successful instructor should be able to keep the pace in working with the children. So if you have decided to be an exquisite and unique children yoga instructor, first of all you need to work on your energy level. This also has a perfect effect on your own personality and lifestyle; In fact remember that this doesn't mean you have to put too much pressure on yourself or compromise yourself but to keep a positive mind and a joyful and lively state of energy.

-If you find that children enthusiastically attend the class, set your goal as to maintain this enthusiasm. In training children, we should make a balance between what we teach them and what they want to learn. The right way to hold each yoga class session in the most positive way possible is to let them express their creativity within the class facilities.

-As mentioned before, yoga cannot be conveyed to children the way it is conveyed to adults. So, what is the appropriate method? Since "playing" is the most interesting topic for any child, we use interesting and creative games to convey different concepts and instructions to them. Why not! Have you ever played with children? Do you remember your childhood? If your playmate doesn't have an active presence during a game, your passion will surely diminish. So if you want to maintain children's enthusiasm in the games and during your class, you should enjoy the game yourself first.

Children are creative, and if they are not suppressed but encouraged instead, they are not afraid of creating new worlds. One way to attract children is to hold a variety of creative classes. Work on your creativity; However, working with children of different ages automatically affects your creativity. Go to nature and get inspired by it; Mother Nature is the fountain of beautiful phenomena and inspirations. Don't limit your imagination and allow your mind to fly.

- The way you speak in the class is of great importance. Talking monotonously distracts playful children easily. Don't shout but don't be monotonous and hypnotic either. Practice raising or lowering your voice at the time. Being successful in conveying any sense is highly dependent on how you speak. Practice being impressive. Remember that long pauses in speech as well as talking too much make children bored and weary.

- Be prepared each time that the schedule may not go the way you expected. Be flexible and enjoy change. Go with the energy of children and don't get upset if the class won't turn out as you planned!

- Children are too straightforward; Practice to increase your ability to hear. Be aware of your emotions. You should work on yourself to be confident so as not to be irritated by their words. They express themselves easily. For example, they may say: "How yellow your teeth are! You're obese, you're ugly… and things like this.

In such cases, avoid harsh and violent reactions. Accept yourself the way you are and practice accepting others the way they are. When you have a good relationship with yourself, your students also want to be like you. Accept that you are not supposed to be pleasant and loveable to everyone. Just be yourself and let those around you be comfortable with who you are, as you are. One of the most important points when working with children is the instructor's mental preparedness. So, work on yourself correctly.

- Be up to date. Being up to date with the world of children is of a great significance. Watch new cartoons and animations and get updates about any trends in computer games or applications kids use and play and also get to know children's favorite characters and songs. Sometimes you can use cartoon space to make a better and closer connection with them. It also makes children trust you and accept you as a person with similar interests as theirs.

- Do not discriminate between children. They feel it well. Take the same look at all of them and teach them this look. They learn from you that we are all like each other, and no one is superior to another.

- Be careful in connecting with boys and girls. You cannot make a relationship with a tough boy with pink color, flowers, fairies or talking with a childish tone and expect him to take you seriously. However, you can teach them that all colors and tastes are beautiful, and it's okay if a boy likes pink or a girl likes blue!

- The important thing is to remember you are not a psychologist or psychoanalyst, but you just spend some impactful moments of teaching yoga to kids in a safe, happy and enjoyable environment.

- If you encounter a child with mental health problems in your classroom, you should discuss the problem in a few meetings with his parents, considering their capacity and mental readiness, and offer suggestions for improving the situation. If you take the problems of each child home with you, you will seriously get hurt over time. Know that through yoga you will have positive effects on them, and over time positive changes will be achieved.

-**Now:** I propose that you pick up a pen, a piece of paper, and write down your motivations for working with children; why do you want to teach yoga to children? What are the strong points you feel in yourself in this regard? Or what are the weak points you should work on for your success?

An accurate knowledge of purpose and motivation greatly helps you to find the right path and move on it.

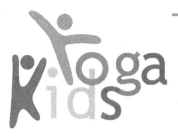

CHAPTER 3
Inner Child healing

"In every real man a child is hidden that wants to Play".
Friedrish Nietzsche

"Inner Child" is the intact and real part of each person.

All of us experience different things in childhood or even adolescence due to our inability to make decisions and choices, on which we have no control. Each of these events affects our soul, mind, and emotions, and forms various feelings in us. Of course, we are now able to make our own choices and about past events, we cannot change the past, what we do is that we can choose how to feel about it. For one who works with children it is very important to have an awake and alive, healed child within themselves, because if we make a better relation with our own inner child, we would definitely be more comfortable and understanding with other children. Note that the awakening and healing of the inner child doesn't mean to behave childishly or speak in a childish tone, but is to be real in behavior, become our authentic self and easy in expressing your inner feelings. As a children yoga instructor, you may face children who trigger and challenge emotions that have been repressed deep down your unconscious mind since your childhood. This can even make it difficult for you to continue your work with kids as you will face lots of emotional charges! This is where you need to understand more about yourself. If you have trust into the Universe and the path on which you are walking toward growth, you would know that all the hurts and wounds you suffered from as a child were all necessary to get you to the point where you are now, and made you who you are today. Things can be difficult and stressful in their time and circumstances, but if you pay conscious attention to the events happening to you and meditate on it, you take the lesson, heal the wounded child in you and become more conscious and aware in your path of life.

This is the time when you let go of your role of a victim, happily and joyfully hug your inner child and tell it: "Everything is going to be great, I am with you and you can trust me. From now on, you are my priority and I'm going to take care of you". Have a conversation with your inner child. Ask about its expectations, listen to it, and trust it like it trusts you. If you listen to your inner child, meaning to listen to that little inner voice in your own heart, you'll make more conscious choices and avoid putting yourself into hurtful circumstances. The little child in you, knows what you need for being happy and living a life aligned with the Joy of your soul. And this is where your choices change forever.

As long as you are happy with yourself, you make those around you feel better.

I prepared an audio to support you in your process of "Healing your inner child".

To get access to this guided meditation audio for "Healing the inner child", please visit my website and get a Free access.

www.nobiehkiani.com

> *I believe that if you can introduce yoga to children in a way that they will choose it over any other activities they have the choice of, then, you'll be able to teach any age after that, as you will connect to anybody's inner child and you will find yourself with a gift of a compassionate heart which brings a sense of trust and love in whichever space you step in...*

Enjoy the journey!

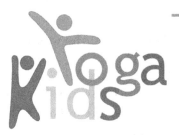

CHAPTER 4

Practical Information for Instructing Yoga to Children

The question that arises here is which yoga asanas are suitable for children and which are not?

Children in different age groups are very different. In this book, different games have been designed for different age groups. Therefore, you can choose the right games based on their level of growth and physical maturity. Of course, a child's age alone doesn't tell everything about him. A six-year-old child may have the experimental age of that of a 4-year old one, or vice versa. When dividing children into separate groups, make sure that you choose the right level of experiment, social relationships, and physical strength.

Divided Age groups

Children between 3 and 5 years old:

Preschoolers usually learn how to use their surroundings and enjoy their activity and movement. Through play, they explore the space around them and are intoxicated discovering their physical potential. They learn how to hop, stand on one leg, blink, run, walk back and forth, hobble, do funny movements and….

For this age group, yoga should include full body movements; movements that are easy to understand. It's important to avoid correcting preschoolers while doing yoga postures.

At this age, children have an amazing imagination power which is quite noticeable in their games; a power that can be used in yoga games. Participating in children's excitement, participating in their fantasies and games, stimulating exploration and understanding their pleasures are among the responsibilities of a yoga instructor. Children at this age move easily but get tired soon. Exercise should be short and enjoyable to make them preserve their energy and concentration.

They enjoy repetition. For example, if you start and end the class with a poem in one session, they may enjoy repeating that poem in each session. Young children often become attached to their parents or nurses and are often conservative about playing with others. Through simple exercises such as holding each other's hands, you may teach them that cooperating with others could be interesting. Talking the language of a puppet you take with you to the class can help them to learn and pay attention. It is better not to talk to them in a childish voice and leave it to your doll. Don't forget that explanations should be absolutely simple and clear.

Children's desire to learn at this age is very high, and at the same time, they can easily get baffled and confused. Time has no meaning for them which may be problematic and boring for you as an instructor because the class time is limited, and you have to get positive results at the end of the class. One solution might be to tell the children at the beginning of each class the program and tasks that are intended for that session, and repeat it throughout the class so that everything goes on according to the plan.

A very important point is that children at this age have a very soft skeleton. Reverse and twisted postures can stretch this skeleton and might be damaging to their bodies. In such exercises, the emphasis is mostly on being very mindful in using the asanas which are adaptable for their bodies. Instead of physically correcting the postures of these children, it is enough to mirror them; do the right posture and remind them to adjust the posture with your guided words. Remember that Warrior Group asanas are better not to be trained for this age group, because they still don't know how to control back muscles, thus may damage their lumbar vertebrae.

Children between 5 and 8 years old:

Children at this age are stronger and have more control on their movements. Physically they are somehow indefatigable and learn more easily. They gradually begin to diversify. This means for an instructor, for example, to avoid repeating a poem in successive sessions. At this age, children use their imagination to discover emotions and accept different roles. For them, it is usually impossible to distinguish between imagination and reality. They still like fantasies, but it is better to get a little closer to reality. Imaginary magic becomes so vivid and real to them that may become a scary truth. As an instructor, keep this in mind. For example, if during the class you are teaching a movement named "Shark", it is best to explain to them that according to the rules of the class, our shark is friends with all the children of the yoga world, or you may even get help from famous cartoon characters whom they like.

Strength, agility, and independence is growing more in them each day, and their abilities are increasing day by day. Sometimes, it is hard for them to understand the right time to stop. As an instructor, you should help them to recognize their limitations, and be careful not to over-stretch their bodies, not overdo and not to hurt themselves. They have full confidence in their instructor and are not aware of the potential dangers. This is upon you to provide their security. At these ages, teaching asanas makes more sense. It is a good idea that you teach them a few basic tips, and then show them the correct posture; then ask them to stay a few breaths after doing the right posture. You can start teaching the Warrior Group asanas with caution and control. At these ages too, you have to correct them with verbal explanations and demonstrating the correct posture, better not to use hands on adjustments.

Basic friendships form at these ages; the child learns how to cooperate and pay more attention to others. Doing partner or group postures further strengthen this feeling in them. Abstract concepts such as freedom, security, loss, and forgiveness find meaning in this period. Some of the games mentioned in this book deal with such concepts.

Children between 8 to 11 years old:

At this stage, the child is separated from his fantasy world. He no longer wants to pretend to be someone but wants to experience it himself. Although home still means security to him, the real world is outside the home; he will enjoy more outdoor activities over time. In the yoga class, children at this age are more likely to seek change, and hardly enjoy imaginary games. This age group is the best time to learn the right techniques. At this stage, they even become smarter than adults, they can perform a variety of postures, and speed is the equal to pleasure. They love to show off and be the best in everything. It is the instructor's job to make the best of the children's, guide and encourage them and at the same time, invite them to rest when needed (for example when there is a danger and the kid is unaware of it). Teach them that yoga is not competitive. The goal of yoga is to increase self-awareness and experience the joy and pleasure of the movements, not to compete and find who's more flexible or stronger! Children who try to get ahead of others usually hurt themselves. Remember not to constantly correct a particular child or constantly remind a student of his behavior, because this way you instill in them a sense of badness or helplessness. It is best to articulate the group as a whole or, if necessary, correct a particular child with a small touch.

At this stage, "friendship" is of great value; the child wants to be different from the others, and at the same time be a part of the group. The age when boys speed up their bikes, and gradually the sense of femininity awakens in girls. At this time, children gain lots of information through various mass media, peer groups and educators. This causes children to often come up with ideas that will surprise their parents. They begin the long journey of change from childhood to puberty!

Some Tips on How to Teach Yoga to Teens:

At this age period, you might face a group that is most insecure and irritable and critical. If you want to take them with you, you have to present everything so-called "cool", otherwise, they won't take you seriously!

To work with this age group, you shouldn't have a childish tone when explaining asanas or games. Try to be yourself.

At this age, comparison becomes more frequent. Curiosity about one's gender and the opposite sex increases. Beauty standards become more prominent. Their self-esteem is usually lowered, and their internal challenges are increased. You should talk to them a lot. Sharing emotions in the class, although they are not willing to do it at first, can be a very important and effective part. It's more interesting to them to do asanas in a cycle. Reverse postures and back-bends are very necessary and useful for improving self-confidence and courage, also since they are very hunched over at this age, postures for opening the heart and shoulders can be so effective.

Games titled "Trust and Cooperation" can be the best option for this age group. Also, creative games are greatly recommended, because by cultivating creativity you help them discover their hidden inner talents and easily find their way in the near future.

"Yoga Nidra" or guided meditation is excellent for them. At this age, Yoga Nidra may take up to 15 minutes. Illustrating, saying positive sentences, and strengthening self-belief are very fruitful. Another important point in working with the adolescent age group, is the trainer's self-mastery and self-confidence. They taunt you or you may even be ridiculed. This behavior is usually caused by a lack of self-confidence. All you must do is to be confident and work on yourself. The common rules must be taken seriously, straightforward, and orderly, as well as being run in the class, otherwise classroom management can become challenging!

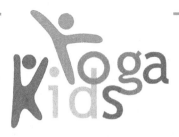

CHAPTER 5

Basic Principles of Teaching Yoga to Children: Instructor's role

The instructor plays an important role to guide the yoga games. They must be supportive & encouraging at the same time.

- Don't put them under any pressure. Ask them in a friendly way to do the exercises. If they are naughty or get tired fast, ask them for their explanation. This shows respect.
- Pay positive attention to them. Help them to understand that everyone has different powers, ability, and talent. Emphasize the non-competitive side of yoga. Children should enjoy the exercises. Discourage laughing at others who are not doing the exercises 'correctly'. Remind that everyone should do it in their own way with their own abilities.
- Make them understand clearly about your expectations during a class. Children like honesty. If there is any behavior that you don't like, warn them gently and let them know. Talk to them in their own language.
- Create a relaxing atmosphere to start the class. If the children are coming directly from school, you can start the class with a glass of juice or mineral water. It will help them talk about the things that happened during their day or even about the last session.
- Respect their opinions. Most often children bring interesting subjects. Allow them to express themselves.

- Help them know each other better in a group. Start the class by asking them to sit in a circle and say their names loudly. Or each child can invent a movement presenting themself to the group.

- Older children can invent a movement with their own names. You can make the "Name Game" sound like a story. For example: "My name is Sarah, I am going on a trip." As the game is going on in the circle, each child must put the name of the one before, in their story. Do your best to encourage them to remember each other's names. Once they remember each other's names, they will feel better connected.

- SAFETY: Keep potentially dangerous items like sharp objects and jewelry away. Inform them that eating or chewing anything is dangerous while practicing.

- Ask them to use the toilet before the class. otherwise for example: 'Can I use the toilet please?' Sarah asks. Then the rest will follow! and you end up kids constantly asking to have a go!

- Encourage friends to find their independence. Some games are for pairs, and you may find certain couples always want to work together. Keeping the same partner is limiting because children never get the chance to discover different peoples' ideas and styles. Discourage this by forming couples randomly through different methods. Try to keep "friends" from always sticking together.

- Remind them to laugh with each other, not AT each other. Sometimes children just feel giggly and want to spend the class time laughing at random things. If they start to laugh at each other's mistakes, clothes, and so on, this can be hurtful. Help children turn giggling into a fun game in which everyone is included. For example, if they are laughing at someone's socks, you can say: "It's great that their socks made you so happy, have you seen my new silly T-shirt?" After they stop laughing at your shirt, ask each child to find a funny thing in themselves to make everybody laugh. Then say: "Giggling is great when we do it all together. It's not nice if people think you're making fun of them. We can all enjoy laughing together."

- Teach them to pay attention to you and each other. Sometimes they must demonstrate a movement to others, encouraging them to support each other. It's very exciting for them. Some feel shy or scared to demonstrate in front of the class, tell them: "Pay attention so that when it's your turn, others will pay attention to you. Keep smiling and give positive attention to support your friends. It helps people express their ideas without being shy."

- Make sure they understand that some exercises need to be done in silence. You might introduce the relaxation exercises by saying, "In the next few minutes try to be very quiet so that you can feel and see inside yourself. After the exercise is over invite them to share their experience."

- Make use of children's energy; don't try to repress them. You need to be very flexible in your planning. Be prepared to change your lesson plan at any time to match the children's energy. Sometimes a group will be very talkative, giggly and restless so you might let them move freely for a while, and then have each kid think up a movement for the class to imitate. If they need to, let the children run around and release their excess energy at the beginning of class. If this happens in the middle of class, try to do more active yoga poses or play a game.

- Limit the class size to 12 children.

- For children over 6, ask at the beginning of the class if anyone has any physical challenges or pains today. A friendly way to do this is to sit in a circle and have each participant say their names and how their body feels today. Another way is to say "magic" instead of "pain" or ask them if there is anything their body is trying to tell them today.

- Move to another pose, game, or topic if the children lose interest.

- Be patient and try never to be angry, scared, or frustrated. When they see this kind of weakness their negative behavior increases. Arrive with lots of self-confidence, a light heart, and lots of excitement and joy.

- Children watch our behavior and sense subtle feelings. If you respect yourself, they will respect and listen to you.

- Know your students. You can use a questionnaire at the beginning of term or the class session, asking about their favorite animal, color, food, yoga pose, etc. That way you could give them a balloon the color they like or dedicate the pose of a certain animal to them. You will also be able to use their favorite pose in order to draw their attention back to the class if they become distracted.

- Avoid negative words like, "No you can't, impossible, not like that, wrong, don't do"...Instead use positive substitutes like please..."You can do it, can you do it please, maybe you should try this way, I know you can do it," etc.

- Everybody makes mistakes and gets confused sometimes, making it a positive experience.

- Think before you speak. Use simple and clear instructions. Be aware that children are not always sure of right and left. Use "to one side" and then "to the other side." Or you can have them wear a bracelet on the right hand and say, "the side with/ without the bracelet".

- Don't stay in one place. Move around and mix with kids.

- Demonstrate the poses and practice with the kids. They will always imitate your actions rather than follow your words. In poses where the kids cannot see you completely like Plough, Spider, Candle pose etc, demonstrate the pose before guiding everyone into it.

- Use the children to demonstrate poses sometimes. Make sure that you use someone different every time so that everyone gets the same amount of attention. With new groups, it's better to ask for a volunteer rather than to bring everyone's attention to someone who is shy and might be intimidated.

- Ask the kids to help you remember the name of the pose or how to do it, organizing the classroom at the beginning and end of class, and in giving out certain props or prizes.

- Treat all the children equally. The principle of fairness and equality is very important to them.

- Kids should repeat the poses as many times as they want and hold them for as long as they wish to.

- To help the children stay longer in the poses use lots of songs, counting, and sound effects. Sometimes you will need to guide them with instructions like "Higher! Lower! Faster! Deeper! Further!..." to help them stay in the posture for more than just a few seconds.

- Don't hide your physical limitations from kids, so that they know that it is OK if they can't do everything exactly, or if they are not able to do a pose.

- Don't force anyone to participate. If a child is not prepared to join in, let them sit and watch until they feel ready to participate.

- Children are curious about sex. You may come across children who regularly touch parts of their body or ask questions about it in the class. In such cases, it is important that the instructor stay calm and does not get disturbed. This is absolutely normal. If they repeat the practice, you should properly raise the issue with the parents if they are mentally prepared. Otherwise, they may suppress the child's natural sense of sexuality by their misbehavior. If it's not the case, you may talk to the child in private, tell them that it is not appropriate to do it in the class and simply ask him not to do it again.

- It's better not to use music on a regular basis throughout the session in the class, because it may become a run-out-of-the-mill concern. It is best to play music at the right time to have more effect.

- It is better to have yoga mats with the same color, so that kids don't get caught up in having a particular color. But if not, you can use games that make children run around the circle and randomly pause in a mat. This will help in situations where they insist on having a special place such as sitting next to the coach or on a mat with a certain color. This way, without realizing it, their attention is distracted from the mat and other related issues during the game.

- If you praise a child by saying a phrase like "You are the best", definitely explain that anyone can be their best, and no one is superior to others. Children who have received too much attention in the family may become boastful when hearing the sentence "you are the best". On the other hand, children who have been neglected in the family may refuse to believe you and distrust the whole thing. But when we say we are all one, we move together and each of us has to be their best, they stop comparing themselves to others.

- If there is a child in your class who is constantly trying to get attention, you shouldn't let him get all your attention. Look into his eyes and say: No!!! Remind him of the rules, give him indirect attention and continue your program. By giving small signs such as a gesture, snapping, using a talking doll or mentioning a rule such as "only the one who has the talking ball can talk and not anyone else…" make him calm and concentrated.

- "Comparing" happens too often in children above 6 years old. It is good to remind them by using cartoon characters like Shrek (the Green Kind Giant), that everyone has their own beauty. This way you can neutralize the effects that the fashion world and society have on their psyche, to some extent. Inspire them that all creatures are beautiful and loveable exactly the way they are.

- Empathizing with children can be a very significant help in convincing them. For example, when they won't let go of a blanket they took in class with them, you can say: "I know how you feel. I also have a blanket which I like so much and it is so difficult for me to get away from it, but I put it somewhere safe until I get back to it."

- In a fight between two children, it is best to explain the situation first, rather than thinking of punishment. You should encourage them to accept each other's apologies. First let them know why it's not okay to behave as they do. Make them both seated and open the issue, regardless of who is guilty. Ask them some questions and try to solve the problems with their help.

- Sometimes children between the ages 3 and 5 don't come to the class alone and want a parent to be with them. In such cases they can be accepted for a few sessions with their mother or father or a trusted companion to gradually get used to the classroom space.

- All competitions have a winner, but reward your students only when they have done something positive, not when they win a competition. This way, they will understand that they would be rewarded for their appropriate positive behaviors.

- It is better not to use a mirror in the class, since a mirror reflects energy and causes distraction.

- When doing reverse postures or any complicated and advanced postures and asana, tell them that in order to maintain more security and prevent dangerous events it is better for them to use your help and ask them to do the postures only under your supervision.

- A children yoga instructor can prevent the potential physical and bodily problems or even correct children's bodies with the right use of asanas, thus has a positive impact on their lives. So be serious and diligent in teaching asanas correctly.

- Memory cards can play an important role in conducting the class in many sessions. These cards contain a series of images; distributed in two identical sizes. You may simply buy these cards from bookstores or make them yourself. But how can these simple cards help you? Sometimes children don't stay on their own mats, thus a quarrel happens over a special mat. In games that are played in pairs, you constantly have problems choosing playmates…!

  Here, you can use memory cards. Put as many cards in the middle as the number of students or scatter them randomly. The two students who have the same image, become one group. Or if there is a problem over the mat, you may put some cards on the mats and give the rest to the children. They search among the cards on the mats and try to find the same image as they have. Then they sit on the mat with the identical picture as theirs. It is just that a lot of irrelevant disputes will be solved during games.

- Respect a child who wants to skip his turn in a game or a task. Pressure may end in tears. Tell them you will reserve their turn for them when they are ready.

- Give them something to take home, like a sticker, stamp, balloon, etc. They love to have something to show the parents and tell them about their great yoga class. Instead of regular prizes, you can also give them a little colorful note with a positive affirmation on it. You can let the children pick their own gifts from a special goodbye sack.

- Give something special to the children at the end of term, like a diploma, medal, yoga cards, their own pictures, etc…especially if you have been working with the group for the whole year.

- Try to create a connection with the parents. This helps build a community between families and kids, perhaps leading to long lasting friendships.
- **Open your mind, clear your heart, play like a kid, laugh a lot and have fun!!!**

Rules:

Whatever rules you choose to set in your class, make sure you stick to them. Otherwise, children will quickly learn that your rules can easily be broken without consequences and you will have a very hard time managing your class.

Personally, I don't have any strict rules in my classes because I believe that if the class is fun and interesting and appropriate to the age and level of the students, there will be no space for disruptions. Bad behavior is usually just a way of trying to get attention.

To make it fun and set your class rules in a non-strict way, You can use some colorful papers and ask the children to draw and write down the rules themselves and you will put them in a board on the wall so that any time you need, you can refer to the rule and values of your classroom and bring a discipline which is more like a mutual agreement between you and your students for the class to be as productive, fun and pleasant as possible.

Here are a few suggested rules:

- No violence toward oneself or others.
- Listen to your body.
- When one person speaks (whether it's the teacher or a student) everyone listens.
- There's no wrong way to do it!
- You can speak during the class but only with permission.
- Stay on your mat.
- Yoga mats stay on the floor.
- No laughing at each other but laughing together.
- Final relaxation is a quiet time.
- You get what you get, and you don't get upset.
- The rule of "3 Reminders and the quiet Mat": each child receives one reminder card each time they break the rule, If they get 3 reminder cards, must pass one round of the game on a mat, named "quiet mat" and wait until they can join again this time respecting the mutual agreements we set as rules on the board.

Ways to praise

We all like to be admired and praised. We all need to feel successful, respected and acknowledged. Giving children a good feeling about themselves is one of your duties as an instructor, which can be done by paying attention to their positive behaviors and their participation in the class. The more you admire your students, the more enthusiastic they become in the class.

Praise generously, look them in the eye, call them by their name, and mention their specific achievement. Remind them of the special thing they were admired for. Transmit your admiration right at the moment when they do something good which is a positive and kind attention they showed in the class, and make sure you are admiring the behavior which you like to see most in children.

Here are some suggestions for verbal admiration. These sentences must definitely be expressed along with a lot of excitement.

- I'm so proud of you.
- You can do it!
- You got it!
- That's perfect!
- Good going!
- That's the way!
- You are so creative!
- I wish I could do it like you.
- Terrific
- You really perfected...pose.
- You are getting so much better at...
- That's awesome – you figured it out!
- Hey, let's all try to do it like...does.
- That's a great...pose
- You are doing great!
- Wow!
- That's the greatest idea I've ever heard!
- That's the best...pose I've ever seen!
- You are so much fun!
- You are the best group ever!
- I love it when you do...!

- Look at…he/she is doing an amazing…pose!
- Let's give a big hand to…!
- Follow your dreams! Together we can make this world a better place!
- Thanks for waiting your turn!
- Thanks for helping me clean up!
- Other non-verbal ways to praise may be:
- Eye contact
- Smiling
- Nodding
- Thumbs up
- Clapping
- High five
- Laughing
- Hugging
- Patting on the back
- Imitating
- Letting them choose a pose or activity

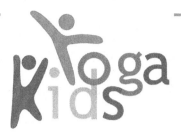

CHAPTER 6
Challenging Children
and how to behave?

Imagine you have started one of your children's yoga classes. You have spent energy and time for a few days to design an interesting schedule for that day. The only thing you don't need at this moment is an aggressive child who enters the class angrily and spoils the class program, ignoring all the hard work you did with love. He throws things away, refuses to play, hurts and annoys other children or worst of all, insults, disrespects or ignores you. This situation is definitely not pleasant and not any instructor will like to face a situation like that! but the reality is that you might encounter a challenging child like that in one of your classes and what makes you a special and different instructor is your ability and skills to deal with the conflict in a mindful and compassionate way. If you fight back or have conflicts with such a child, either the conflict escalates or in the most optimistic case, the child gets calm at the moment and apparently follows the class, but you have not been able to have a profoundly positive impact on his character; By suppressing his feelings, you may probably mislead him in understanding his own feeling. Definitely, such a space is not the goal you were supposed to achieve in working with children. I know this well; if not, you wouldn't be reading this book right now. Before I present the solution, pick up a piece of paper, a pen, and write down the potential solutions you think might be helpful in such cases. Who knows?! maybe you yourself know the right solution from within yourself. Here, I present an exercise for you to understand the issue more clearly. To make children understand their own feelings, you must have experienced and understood these feelings beforehand. First of all, you have to become the same child, and see the world from his perspective. Now, ask a friend, a colleague or anyone who likes working with children to accompany you in the following exercise. Of course, you can do the exercise in a group as well. Here, in this chapter the challenging characters you may face during the class are presented.

We are going to roll play these different characters and come with answers about how to deal in a situation like that!

Plan a sample yoga class together with your friends who join you for the role playing.

One plays the role of a child (choose from the list below) and one as the instructor of that child. Before starting the play and enter into your role, close your eyes for a few moments and put yourself in the place of that child by a few deep breathings. If you play the role of an angry child, fully imagine that you are a child who is carrying a lot of anger; A child who is involved in a conflict with other children, family and parents, or the loss of something you loved too much or the failure of the favorite game.

After you fully get what this character feels at the moment and the emotions aroused in you, now you can open your eyes and according to the role you play enter the game and become the student who participates with those related feelings…

In this section we are going to introduce you into different problematic children behavior you might encounter.

Then, you will see 2 different attitudes an instructor can perform in dealing with the situation.

The wrong one which is not constructive and just suppresses the feelings and complicates the situation for both sides and the right way of dealing with the situation which makes a difference and is with understanding and compassion.

The person who plays the role of the instructor will behave in the two models presented below. The wrong way of reacting and the right way of handling the situation.

The aim of this practice is to understand the child and why he might behave the way he does and make him understand that you are there to support him and not to judge him for who he is.

By explaining the situation you make the child know that he is not a bad person but what he does might be harmful thus you are inviting him as a friend to behave in a way which is friendly and collaborative with you and other kids involved.

*Remember that the category of characteristics presented here are general examples to indicate the behaviors of a child in class and how you can deal with it. NEVER label a child

directly with any adjective as such, but just recognize the behavior and help the child to understand why it is wrong.

NOW,

Go to the list below and play the game with your friends.

Write down in your notebook about your experiences and insights.

Some suggested practices and games such as (dealing with anger and…) are pointed out and represented later in the related chapter.

Angry child:

<u>Wrong attitude:</u>

"Be quiet. Calm down. You look so grumpy again! You have no right to behave like this. Stop it. You are walking on my nerves. Don't shout. Get out of the class. I don't want to hear anything!!"

<u>Correct attitude:</u>

"It seems that you are angry about something today. I understand, sometimes I get angry at certain things too. Now ask the other children: "Guys, have you ever been too angry? I usually feel my anger in my hands, how about you? Would you like to say, one by one, where you feel your anger?", and after everyone comments, you may say: "How amazing. It was different for each of us." Now if you have been taught how to overcome anger in previous sessions, you may tell the angry child: "What do you think? We can, like previous sessions, shake like a jelly and let this anger out, we can partly empty the air like a balloon, or we can roar like a yoga lion pouring out our anger and continue playing our interesting games." And if you haven't still taught them, you may dedicate the same session to teaching how to deal with anger, emptying and directing it.

You will see that the child gets calm and gradually changes his attitude, because you and his friends helped him to overcome his weird feelings.

Inattentive child:

<u>Wrong attitude:</u>

"Sarah, are you listening to me? Do you even hear me? I am talking to you. Listen up! It is very rude that you don't answer! Why don't you play? Am I not talking to you?! You are completely out of the picture! How could you be this much careless? If it is so, please don't play!"

Correct attitude:

You had better draw the attention of such a child indirectly, than to insist on her active presence. For example, say: "Sarah, this is what we are doing. Would you like to participate in the game?" If she is still inattentive and careless, tell her: "It is all right, you can stay out of the game this time, if it's not so interesting to you." Then try to add some excitement to your program, and provoke her a little bit, until she is attracted to the class and draws her attention to you. For example, you may tell the children in a quiet and mysterious voice: "Guys, please gather for a moment, I want to tell you a secret that has to be kept between us. OK?"

If she is still wandering around in the class inattentively and indifferently, it's better to remind her of the rules, and offer to quietly spend some moments on the quit mat until she feels she is interested in the class. Remember, the more you insist such a child, the less she tends to follow either the class or the game. It's a good idea to let go a little and let her move on to the class process. Such a child needs more excitement to be encouraged. She probably thinks the class is boring and insipid. Try to change such a mindset by being more passionate and creative yourself in the classroom.

Crying child:

Wrong attitude:

"Oh, My! This needs no crying. You shouldn't cry. Clam down. Nothing has happened; Take this doll; look it is laughing! Crying is so childish! Don't be a cry baby!

If it is a boy who cries, The man doesn't cry! Come play and you will forget – look we are enjoying. All right, cry as much as you want. Come to class when you finish crying."

Correct attitude:

"Oh! It's as if someone here is upset about something (understanding the child). I understand dear. I know you are upset about it. You have the right to cry (sympathy). Well, you know? I miss someone too, I sometimes cry a lot when someone is bothering me (give an example of your crying experience the way it is comprehensible to them)." Then look into her eyes and say: "What do you think if we wipe away our tears and take a deep breath." If the child is crying out of missing the family, a pet or a toy, tell her: "I can tell you that after the class, you will see X again and your sadness will fade to a great extent. Now that you are here, would you like to participate in the game? This way time goes faster?" If none of these ways helps you calm the child down, leave her alone for a while, stop insisting and wasting other children's time. Every minute or two with a sign of hand or eye you can ask her if she wants to enter the game or not. If the answer is still "No", leave her alone and don't give your whole attention to one child.

Spoiled child:

<u>Wrong attitude:</u>

"Come on, who do you want to complain about again? You're such a little Brat! Why are you gulping like spoiled children? It's not always about you! You are grown up! Don't act like a baby. Defend yourself and don't complain about everyone all the time! It didn't hurt, nothing happened…", or: "Oh! Can't you do this all by yourself? Wait, I get it for you. I do it for you. You come and sit with me!"

<u>The correct approach:</u>

"Hmm…it seems that you are upset with Sam? Sometimes it happens during the game. I saw he didn't mean it. I think it was an accident. Would you like to come back to play? I know it hurts. I feel pain in this movement too. You may do it more slowly if it is very painful. Sweetie, I know you are upset but take a few breaths and try to stop crying so that I can hear you; when you cry I cannot understand what has happened, explain it to me."

Or if he refuses to do something that you know he can do alone, tell him: "You can do it; I know you can make it; I want you to try."

Narcissist child:

<u>Wrong attitude:</u>

"Oh yes, your clothes are very pretty! Of course, you are the most beautiful girl! You are the strongest boy in the world! What beautiful hair you have. How sweet you speak, etc.

Or: "It is not good to brag about yourself this much! Stop showing off! Don't think you are better than others. Don't watch yourself in the mirror this much."

<u>Correct attitude:</u>

"Yes, Sam, I see that today your shirt has such a nice color. Guys, do you see how amazing Tom's hat is today? Look at John's bag; it has an extra pocket in which so many things can be placed." Also find an interesting point for praise and attention in all children. You can tell them all, and not to a particular child: "All of us are beautiful the way we are. We are all the best of ourselves. Everyone has a characteristic that is very good and valuable. All of us are God's creatures. No one is superior or inferior to others."

Restless child:

<u>Wrong attitude:</u>

"Sit still for a moment. Don't move this much. Can't you stay still? No, it is wrong. Don't move your legs this much. Why can't you stop? Get back to your mat. Don't you calm down and settle? Enough! you are spoiling the game. You better go to the quit mat; I don't know how to calm you down!"

<u>Correct attitude:</u>

"Well, it's like someone has lots of energy today (call their name and draw their attention to you). Sarah has lots of energy today. What do you think? let's dance and jump for a while before we get into the game. I have exciting music. I guess you may enjoy it. Let's release our energies so we can learn a new game." A restless child needs to release her energy. You cannot expect an energy bomb to keep the order of the game. If there is still no change in her after trying all these methods, making sure that she is not hyperactive, you may remind her of the rules in a determined and sincere manner, rather than angrily and threatening. You can suggest the relaxation mat, or may even put a pillow or cushion on the mat and ask the child to empty her restlessness by tapping on the pillow and return to the game when she is ready to resume play, after letting you know. You may also use this cushion for unloading anger and…

Attention-seeking child:

<u>Wrong attitude:</u>

There are two types of errors here; either pay too much attention to the child looking for attention or ignore her which makes her feel worthless.

"Yes you are right. Yes you are doing well. Oh, Sarah you are marvelous. Yes, come and sit next to me. OK I take your hand. Hmm, deal, we play this game. All right you play first. (… paying too much attention and then getting confused).

or:

No it's enough. No you are the last one to play. Go over there; don't get so close to me. Let others talk too."

Correct attitude:

As mentioned before, first give the child a little attention. But very soon, share this attention among all children. For example, if you already listened to her, now ask other children to take turns in talking in that regard. Or you can listen to her for a while, then looking directly to her eyes, say: "Very well sweetheart, now it is the time for doing this asana or it is now our other friend's turn. Let us talk about it after the class." Or if she tries to sit next to you and play with you all the time, change her place during the game in an indirect way, by using games which need displacement, such as memory cards and…When she is drowned in the game, she automatically joins other children and everything goes on smoothly. Make sure that you give equal attention to all children; don't pay much attention to one child and ignore another.

controlling child:

Wrong attitude:

"You are not the teacher! It shouldn't always be your way! You are a bad girl. You are annoying everyone. You had better stop such behavior. Am I not talking to you? I don't listen to you because you did this. If you want to continue this behavior, you better not be in this class at all!

Correct attitude:

In such cases, you definitely should not pay a ransom to the child, and you should not enter a game of force with her and provoke her further. But, you may deal with her by using words, being determined and reminding the rules: "Well, apparently someone is here today that wishes to sit on the teacher's mat or wants us to play the Mirror Game. Well I know you like this mat or you are fond of this game. I understand, but today we are going to play a variety of interesting games. If you accompany us well, I promise we will play the Mirror Game next week. Or, today Sarah is sitting on this mat and it is not friendly if we make her change her place. But if you come sooner next week, you may be able to take that mat. If she still continues to insist and be restless, tell her: "Well, we have a quiet mat here on which I think you have to sit for awhile and think about my suggestions."

You should express your demand with sincerity and determination, and remind her of the rules. Also, you may direct her strength and power toward a positive task, or get her distracted by playing and dancing games.

Rude child:

Wrong attitude:

In such cases, the child is either blamed too much: "O rude! What an ugly word was that? Didn't they teach you any manners? It was the last time you said that! You've been rude again! You are so mean! Or her behavior is too much denied: "No, Sarah didn't say that, you heard it wrong! Sarah never talks like this. She is a good girl. It slipped off her tongue."

Correct attitude:

In such cases, try to stay calm, cool and determined. Don't get confused. Don't get angry. Look directly into her eyes and say: "Dear Sarah, this word doesn't have a good meaning; if you heard it somewhere, you shouldn't repeat it in the class honey. It's better if you express your request and use other words in the classroom so that we can understand you all and no one gets hurt by the words you use, because I know you really don't mean to say those hurtful words and you never meant to be mean to anyone. We are all a circle of loving friends here and I am your friend too and because I love you I don't want you to also express yourself in a way in which you might not know how you might hurt my feelings by the wrong language you used in mistake!

Then you just repeat again to the child that: Please don't repeat it in this class!

And as an alternative you can suggest that they can use Gibberish language (which is explained in the section of emptying anger) putting our ugly words inside a bag and when our Jiberish swearing is over, put the bag inside the dustbin and continue playing.

Isolated and shy child:

Wrong attitude:

"Oh, don't be shy; come play; come on; children, take her hand; oh, are you ashamed? Don't you want to talk? Say something; come play and you will change your mind; you cannot stay aside; come on here; it's not good to stand at the corner; come on here."

Correct attitude:

Look directly into her eyes and say: "It seems that you are not ready to join us yet! But once you decide to accompany us, rest assured that you can trust me and make yourself comfortable. We start the exercise; come and play with us when you think you are ready. Then without insisting, prepare the class and every minute or two, ask her if she is ready to accompany you in exercises and games with a sign of hand or eye. Give her time to trust you, while she is not being paid attention by other children so much. Remember to give this child a sense of confidence.

Talkative child:

Wrong attitude:

Two wrong things can happen here. One is that you value the child too much, listen to her too much and waste the time of the class and the other children's turns. And the other is that you suppress her and ignore her words. For example: "It is not the time now. Stop please. Let's continue the class. You cannot talk all the time. That's enough. Don't interrupt me over and over. Leave the story for later!

Correct attitude:

In such cases, listen to the child for a while, and then ask her to continue after and outside the class. Like: "Aha, very interesting. I very much like to listen to you dear Sarah, but now is the time for doing exercises" or: "Now it is Mira's turn to talk. Make sure to tell me more at the right time. But now I want you to listen to me or to your friends." Again using Gibberish language could be useful.

Stubborn child:

Wrong attitude:

"No, we do what I say. Now it is not the time for that at all. You had better listen and accompany the class. Stop resisting! Can't you say okay like others just once?"

Correct attitude:

"Dear, I know that maybe this asana is not your favorite one, but inside our Magical Jungle, we need a monkey now! I need you to listen carefully and try to be a funny monkey! Maybe you like it If you do it well. But anyway, know that learning this will help you to perform your favorite posture more accurately. It would be very nice if you accompany me."

Keep in mind that if you pay too much attention to her, her stubbornness will increase. Try to take her with you by giving her responsibility or drawing her attention to a team work: "I want you to help me continue the class."

Eventually, if none of the ways are useful, it is better to keep on going with your class and to not pay any more direct attention to her.

If you practiced all the roles correctly, put yourself in the shoes of each instructor or each child in the mentioned situations, you can now largely understand your feelings as well as the challenging child's. Remember that children don't have bad intentions in their behaviors. Only occasionally do they become involved in their emotions and become confused in recognizing them. If you help them see and understand their feelings, the conflict is over, and the situation is much calmer than you think. Use this practice as often as possible and try to understand the behaviour and come up with the most compassionate solutions.

Ultimately, don't wait for a miracle to happen; be patient and give time to everything.

Some shared experiences of yoga kids ttc trainees during their internship related to kids behaviors applying the suggested solutions:

- Marie explains her experience in one of her classes, as follows:

"In one of the sessions when the trainer invited children to draw a group painting, controversy over the color of markers began, and each child wanted the color the other child had. The trainer decided to hold the markers in hand for each child to pick one by chance with closed eyes; any marker she took would be hers. The result was that the children enjoyed the game and were completely happy with their markers. Amazingly enough, during the painting, they lent their markers to each other during painting without any conflict."

In another experience in inviting children with closed eyes, Marjan describes:

"In one of the sessions, we were dealing with a restless and hyperactive boy who refused to close his eyes for the end of class(savasana). I tried to make the savasana interesting to them by saying that if you close your eyes and look at the black screen in front of your closed eyes, you will see interesting images. Even you would be able to depict images in that darkness." This way I succeeded in encouraging them to keep their eyes closed and accompany me for a while.

Once I happened to come across two restless little boys who performed asanas well and correctly, physically wise. We decided to ask them to show their friends how to perform the asanas properly during the practice. This gave them a boost of energy in order to work with the class and relax. So, the classroom planning continued a regular basis.

Once, there were two little girls named "Claire and Tania". They were so attached to each other that they didn't accept to get apart and both sat on the same mat. Interestingly, both of them sat on a yellow mat, while the only mat which was not taken was another yellow one. The trainer made a smart use of this and told them: "If one of you sits on the other mat, then you both have a yellow mat and are both on the same color mat." It worked. One of them rapidly moved to the other mat and the problem was solved easily.

In one session, two twin sisters named "Roxana and Atena" entered the class. One of them didn't cooperate. She didn't want to enter the classroom, while the other one was busy eating dried sour cherries! We told Roxana, who didn't want to enter the classroom, that she could sit in a corner and join us once she felt ready. She accepted and sat in a corner. Between the games, I pointed to her two times, asking if she liked to join or not. The second time she accepted and joined the class happily, excitedly and confidently. But Atena, who was by no means willing to give up on her sour cherries…The idea that came to my mind at that moment was to tell her that I would make her a paper funnel, put the cherries in it and keep it somewhere for her. Amazingly, she showed interest in the idea and accepted it; so, the problem was solved easily.

- Anita, another intern of the course, describes her experiences as follows:

In a "Name Game" where I asked children to say their names along with their favorite color, when the first one said he liked purple, the others also introduced themselves in purple. When it came to me, I said I like yellow, blue, pink and purple. After that, they one by one declared different colors they liked and stopped imitating one child.

- Dina described her experience as follows:

We had a little girl who liked to sit on the pink mat in every session. From time to time between the games, before she realized, I would sit on that particular mat, and she would have to go to another mat. Then I told her: "Kids, look how Rosha shines on the yellow mat." And of course, after that I told this about all other children with their particular mat color. This gradually lowered Rosha's sensitivity to pink color.

Dina's another experience in a class with eight noisy 9-year-old boys who seemed impossible to calm down, was like this:

"When I found the class so noisy, I asked them to play the "Silent Statues" game. But it didn't work, and they were still mischievous. Then I decided to play the role of a silent statue and let them try to make me laugh. They loved it! and used all their energy trying to make me laugh! I sat still and they tried about 15 minutes to make me laugh but they couldn't. It was interesting to them how calm I was. Then they started playing and tried to sit calm as I did and the class calmed down.

- **Sheri also tells about her experience in using a small doll that she learned about during the course. A doll named Mr. Happy face!**

Sheri explains:

"I had a student who behaved abnormally and constantly tried to express opinions and manners that were associated with violence and negativity, thus disrupted the classroom. Fortunately, using "Mr. Happy face" who I had introduced to children at the beginning of the class, for a few times and talking to them in a different voice as the puppet, I could calm him and make him follow the class."

In another experience, she says:

> "A little girl in the class began to cry after hearing "The Magical Jungle"; she said she was afraid of magic. I told her: "Magic is colorful and beautiful, but if it annoys you, we may call it the Jungle of Dreams!" But she was still crying. Her sister who was with her in class said she was in fact crying for their friends who were playing outside; she liked to go out and play there. I told her: "How do you know? Maybe those who are outside wish to be here in our class and do yoga; you can tell them about our class when you go out." This sentence completely worked, the child calmed down and joyfully joined the game."

And here one of my own favorite stories:

"In one of my after school yoga activities, once I faced a little boy of age 7 who came to class wearing all white. when we started to go through the warmups, He was not doing anything. Just standing there with a grumpy face, folded arms, looking around. I asked him a few times to participate but he wouldn't even answer. Then he started to annoy other kids by bullying or kicking and just acting weird! So when giving him a few notices I realized it wouldn't work,

40

I asked kids to have a few minutes of continuing the warm up without me, making them all responsible to respect the class rules while I took the annoyed kid into another space and spoke to him in private. I explained the situation and how i felt with his reaction and that I care for him and want him to join because I know we can have lots of fun together! Then I asked him what was wrong? The kid hesitated for a bit and told me something which almost made me cry! As we never know what's happening in someone's mind when they are acting in a way which is irritating…He told me that his mother made him wear the white yoga outfit and when he came to the class and saw everyone else wearing colorful and normal clothing, he felt embarrassed and didn't want to take part anymore! At that point, I smiled at him and said oh! This is not something to worry about! Your outfit is perfect! and even if you don't like it, you can imagine you are wearing a superman outfit and feel super powerful! He frowned at first and almost shouted that: THIS IS NOT TRUE AND IT WILL NEVER WORK! I told him yes! Your imagination can create any feeling you want. I'm going to introduce a really fun game now in the class and I'm sure you're going to love it and don't want to miss that! I told him, I leave you here now and you can come back when the magic has worked on you! And I went back to the class. A few minutes later I saw him coming and he shouted in excitement that: IT WORKED! and he joined with lots of enjoyment for the rest of the class and totally forgot about his white outfit!

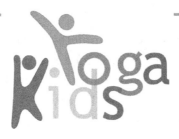

CHAPTER 7
Goals of Yoga Games

As mentioned earlier, the best way to teach yoga to children is through games. Games are used for a specific purpose, and each of them conveys special concepts of yoga.

Children need two things:

1- Deep roots with which they confidently stand on their feet!
2- Wings with which they are able to fly and rise!

Flying alone causes the path to be lost, and root alone destroys the power of imagination. For healthy growth and maturity, children need a safe, supportive, and lovely environment. Their wings for flying in the sky of life grow only when their roots are strong in the ground.

Yoga with its physical and respiratory exercises, can improve self-awareness and self-confidence in children.

The yoga games introduced here help children experience a sense of strength, balance and ultimately a sense of flight.

The goals of these games are as follows:

Creating a strong & healthy body:

The variety of movements offered in the games help children to gain flexibility, strength, balance and endurance. Breathing exercises teach them how to breathe properly, expand the volume of the lungs and increase patience. With relaxation exercises, children learn how to relax their bodies during exercise or work out. You will find out that these games largely help to balance the energy level of children, so after a yoga session, children who are too lively, become calm and relax and at the same time exuberant. Ultimately, many of these games give children a view of their body and how it moves.

-Developing sensory awareness:

Physical recovery helps with mental improvement. Yoga looks at the human as a whole: mind and body are one. Yoga games help children balance their emotions, calm their minds and increase their concentration; they also teach them how to be more adaptable to unexpected events.

With the help of relaxation exercises (sitting in meditation), children learn how to observe their thoughts, and realize that they are something beyond: "beautiful me, ugly me, cowardly me, stupid me, best me". Children can understand their emotions and express themselves in a more compassionate way and become more conscious about their existence; then we can better understand them as well and enjoy their amazing, creative nature as it is.

-Establishing social relationships:

The games that are introduced here are capable of being played in pairs, small groups or even the whole class. Many of the introduced postures are only practicable when children cooperate. They realize that sometimes group work leads to better results than individual work. Doing movements together helps them communicate more with each other, pay more attention to each other, thus become more considerate of others.

In many games, children are asked to invent their own movements and demonstrate them to others. Such games intensify children's self-confidence. They learn how to work with others in the group, while maintaining their individuality.

Developing a sense of creativity:

Many yoga games allow children to create their own movements, immerse in imaginary games, paint and creatively express themselves. These games encourage children to achieve their originality and initiative and use it throughout their lives.

Structuring a class

Each yoga game can be played on its own or in combination with other games.

Different yoga exercises have been divided into these groups:

1. Beginnings
2. Warm up & Ice breaking games
3. Breathing exercises and related games
4. Yoga asanas and related games
5. Sitting exercises and Meditations
6. Group practices
7. Creative games
8. Trust and cooperative games
9. Relaxation

How to structure & design a yoga kid session?

In order to structure and design a yoga session, you can use the map provided below to design your 1 hour and 45 minutes classes suitable for children.

For kids of 6-12 years old, one hour is a suitable time. The session is not too long so that they get tired and it's not too short so that you can have enough time for them to explore the activities and enough time to relax before they leave the session.

For younger kids of age 3 to 5 years old 45 min is enough as they can get tired fast and also a shorter and simpler session for this age group is more effective and easier to digest the ideas.

The way to use the maps is that, You'll come up first with your class theme or subject, after, you can go through different sections in this book to collect some ideas then design your session with the structure as follows below.

It's better you keep the skeleton as it is but be flexible in managing the timings due to your subject and chosen games.

Always go to your class with a prearranged and structured class map but be flexible to change your plan once you find the class capacity or the level of kids energy is different than what you have planned for them.

be prepared and organized, but also be in the moment and use your creativity & imagination to create a unique experience for yourself and kids in your amazing yoga kids sessions.

Assembling and designing a one-hour class for children of 6 to 12 years old:

- 10 minutes beginning
- 10 minutes warm up or ice breaking games
- 10 minutes teaching asana
- 15 to 20 minutes playing games related to introduced asanas
- 5 minutes cool down
- 5 to 10 minutes ending relaxation

Assembling and designing a 45-minute class for children of 3 to 5 years old:

- 10 minutes beginning
- 5 minutes warm up or ice breaking games
- 15 to 20 minutes teaching asana and related games
- 5 minutes cool down
- 5 to 10 minutes ending relaxation

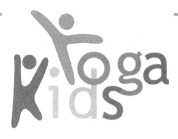

CHAPTER 8
Beginnings

There are many ways to begin the class. If it is a new group, it's better to start with a short introduction about what yoga is, and a name game before moving onto one of the following exercises.

It is good to start the class the same way each time, as it creates a routine that helps kids with discipline. Start by gathering them in a circle with a prayer. Chanting om (see below) is always fun for them and brings more energy to the class. Then you can use the magical sunflower dance, sun dance, mirroring games or any other warms up to start if they come with a high level of energy to your class. Gauge their energy, the last thing you want to happen is for the kids to get bored, both teacher and child will suffer then!

Explaining yoga to children

1- Yoga is a very ancient science that helps us to develop flexibility and strength in our bodies, and happiness and peacefulness in our mind. In yoga, there is a pose for everything in the world, whether it is an animal, a tree, or an airplane, and we can do it with our body.

2- Thousands of years ago, the ancient yogis lived in the forest, the mountains, and caves in India. They observed their environment and saw how animals and nature move in perfect harmony. They imitated the movements of the animals, the trees, the mountains, and even movements of the stars, and created a wonderful technique called yoga.

3- Yoga is a way to exercise our bodies, our breath, and our minds all at the same time. Yoga makes you feel great!

4- Yoga is a practice and philosophy that believes happiness is our natural state. When the body and mind goes out of balance, we do not feel this happiness. With the help of yoga poses, breathing exercises, and focusing within, we bring back this harmony to our body and mind, and come back to this natural state of happiness.

5- For the younger ones, you can use the theme of the magical jungle of yoga. In the jungle, they can find different animals, plants, trees etc. Sitting in a circle like a colorful sunflower, the wind blows, and each petal blows away and turns into different items existing in the magical jungle of yoga! And go on with the story...

Explain OM

Om is the sound of the universe. When God created the universe a vibration or sound came with it and OM is that vibration. The sound of unity, the universe in one sound.

Choose a word: it can be the name of an animal, your name, or the sound of an animal, or anything you like. When you have your word or sound, now everyone chants the chosen sound together! All of those sounds together become OM! (help to wrap it up into a big OM).

You can explain how Om gives an inner massage to your heart and our brain: put one hand on your heart and one hand on the top of your head. Sing OM loudly and feel the pleasant massage the sound gives both to your heart and brain.

For smaller children, you can play this game:

Invite each child to think of something that really surprises them and repeat 'ooooooooooooooooooo!' after each imaginary surprising event.

Next, ask them to think of something yummy! Repeat 'mmmmmmmmmmmmmm!' after each child shares their delicious subject to eat.

Then, join the two sounds together making one sound, 'Ooooooooooooooooooo! Mmmmmmmmmmmmmmmm!'

Suggestions about chanting "OM"

- Oming to each other: sit back to back in pairs and lean together. Take a deep breath and chant "OM" out loud. Feel the vibration of the sound between your hearts.

- Heart "OM": sit in pairs facing each other. Place your hands on each other's hearts from front and behind (like a loop). Repeat "OM". Feel the vibration in the palm of your hands.
- Om circle: sit in a circle, knees touching, and place your right hand over your heart and left hand on your friend's back, right behind the heart. Chant Om out loud and feel the sound opening your heart right in this space between your palms.

Om wave: sitting in a circle, the teacher starts by chanting Om followed by the person to their right. The Om keeps travelling around the circle in this wave form, each participant repeating the sound again when they hear the person on their left doing it again.

Name Games

When you call someone by their own name rather than saying: "Hey you", you give them attention and respect. If someone walks away from the group, the best way to get them back is to call their name and invite them back.

Here are presented some games helping kids to know each other's name also in this way you keep the name of students in mind:

1. Name Ball:

Turn the ball hand in hand as you sit in a circle. Whoever has the ball in hand, it's his turn to speak. You can ask them to say their name along with the name of their favorite animal, color, food, job, yoga asana or….To make the game more attractive, you can pass the ball by foot, instead of passing it by hand.

2. Who is Here Today? (Singing):

The teacher sings: Who is here today?

The child replies: Sarah is here today!

Then all of them sing and dance: "Sit down, jump up, spin in the air, Sarah is here, Sarah is here!"

3. Thankful Ball:

We sit in a circle and pass the ball to each other. Whoever has the ball in hand is saying: "I'…(his/her name), and I'm thankful for…For example: "I am thankful for the sunshine, beautiful flowers, songs of the birds, my wonderful yoga class! etc.

4. Laughter Circle:

Everyone will make a special laugh, and while laughing, say their name, their nationality and their favorite activity. Even if the laughter is not real, the laughing continues; laughing is fun and contagious! You can ask them to make a serious face, then have a fake laugh! It's so funny that it makes everyone laugh!

5. Massage Name:

Sit in a circle with legs wide open, placing their hands on the shoulders of the ones before and after them. Everyone says their name adding the tone and inflection & volume of their voice related to the massage that is being received. If the massage is very gentle, they say their name quietly, and if it is intense, they say it louder. In another method, children can sit behind each other in a queue, like a train but in a circular way so that the first and last person also receive a massage when you change the direction of the queue then they place their hand on each other's back and exchange a massage in the same way.

In this game, you get to know the names of the children as well as receiving a massage!

6. Name and Pose:

Stand in a circle. One child starts by saying her name along with a gesture (it can be a yoga asana or any other movement). Then all children repeat the movement and repeat her name together. The next child who introduces himself should say the name and imitate the gesture of the previous student, then says his own name along with his special gesture. To make this game more attractive, you may make a Vinyasa cycle with the movements children create, or ask them to stay in the movement for a few deep breaths.

7. Traveling Around the World:

Sit in a circle. Saying your name and the name of the student next to you, begin like this: "My name is Sarah, I wish to go to Greece and take Sasha with me." Sasha then goes on to say her name, the name of the country she wishes to travel to and the name of the student before her. The last student should take all the students before her by mentioning their names!

This game improves memory, attention, and concentration, increases the sense of intimacy and familiarity with each other. Meanwhile, you may take a geographical sphere to the class with you so that the children find the country they wish to travel to by rotating the sphere or by their own choice. This way you will also help them to explore their planet earth.

8. Replacement:

Someone introduces herself, moves toward another student and sits in her place; she stands up and after introducing herself, does the same thing with another student, and this goes on until everyone is introduced and replaced.

9. Chanting names:

Using the methods used to chant "OM", each child chants their names and the rest repeat it collectively. This method calms the mind and the vibration of chanting enhances a positive vibe in the classroom. Hearing one's own voice is pleasant and creates a sense of pleasure in their hearts. It also greatly helps to improve stuttering and overcoming shyness.

10. Emotion Circle:

You may begin like this: "Everyone takes turns expressing their feelings at that moment, and at the same time, introduce themselves along with their feelings."

11. Dance Your Name:

Everyone shows their names in Latin letters by making a physical drawing like a dance by creating the letter in their body posture, then others should guess the name.

12. Imaginary Basket:

Imagine there is a basket in the middle of the class. Of course, you may also put a real basket in the class. Everyone says their name and puts something imaginary in the basket according to the subject of the class. For example, if the subject of the class is fruits, ask them to name a fruit as well as introducing themselves, and pretend to put the fruit in the basket. At the end of the class, you may fill the basket with real fruits and invite them to enjoy eating them together.

Ice-breaking Games:

When a class has just begun or one (or more) student has just been added to the class, it usually takes a while for the children to become comfortable and familiar with each other and communicate as they should. Here are some examples of the games that can shorten this time and break the so-called ice between children sooner:

Find the angel Game:

Items needed: Blindfolds

Give everyone a blindfold, ask them to close their eyes and start walking in the class cautiously and slowly. With a secret sign, you choose a child as the angel without letting others notice. For example, you may whisper a word softly in her ear or gently tap her shoulder with a feather or a stick, the way only she understands. The angel stands in her place and doesn't walk. Other children take turns in asking each other slowly: "Are you the angel?!" If the answer is yes and they find the angel, they stick to her and stand there, and if not, they get to others and try as long as they find the angel and become an angel themselves!

Eventually, they all turn into a nice group hug! Now you may ask them to repeat "OM" Mantra together and feel each other's vibrations.

In this game, it's better to avoid placing any device that children may bump into during the practice as they have their eyes closed and you need to make sure that they are all safe in the classroom.

These safe touches, secret communications and group hugs help children get to know each other better and their so-called ice breaks!

Colorful Balls:

Items needed: A number of balls, size of a tennis ball, with different colors.

Place the balls in the middle of the class. Ask the children to stand or sit around the classroom, then by the start of a piece of music, ask them to start collecting the balls, take one ball at a time and place it on their mat. They can continue gathering balls until the music stops. Eventually, each child has a number of balls; some more and some less. Keep up the game so that each of them has at least one ball of each color. For example, if a child has 3 blue balls and another one doesn't have any blue balls, ask them to exchange their balls such that everyone has at least one ball of each color. Now ask them to sit in a circle along with their balls. Each color is a symbol which you have predetermined. Ask the children to take turns in throwing a ball of a particular color, sharing something about the related subject you already introduced, and the color represents.

For example:

Red ball: your favorite hobby
Orange ball: your favorite food
Yellow ball: your dream job
Purple ball: your fear
Blue ball: your best memory
Green ball: your favorite place on the planet

Eventually, everyone shares their thoughts and feelings by throwing the ball in the middle of the circle.

You have a beautiful scene of colorful balls all gathered in the middle of your circle representing all the sharings you had in your circle of friendship.

Naturally this causes more intimacy, warmth, and friendship between children.

Friendship Questionnaires:

Take as many suggested questionnaires to the class as the number of students. If they are illiterate, you may ask them the questions orally. Otherwise, spread them among the children and give them time to fill them in. After they answer all questions, you may play a refreshing gentle music and ask them to walk through the class with their sheets in hand and look at each other's eyes. Every time the music is stopped by you, stand in front of the closest student, and look into each other's eyes for a few moments. Now, everyone takes turns in reading 3 of their answers to the other. Their answers to these questions are nothing but their tastes, decisions, dreams, valuable things or a part of their experiences. By doing so they introduce themselves to each other and share some parts of their lives to each other making them feel close to each other and promote a sense of trust among the group they want to practice with.

Variety of the game: Eventually you may ask children to sit and take turns in sharing their answers with others.

Variety of the game: take the questionnaires from children. From each questionnaire, read a few answers and let children figure out whose questionnaire was that. This makes them pay more attention to their conversation and remember each other. This is nothing but the outburst of friendship and intimacy!

*** Exercise:

You'll find a couple of suggested questionnaires below.

Before you take the questionnaires to the class, first answer them for yourself.

Trust me; you will enjoy discovering the world inside you and thinking about the answers to these questions. Then, hand in a copy of it to a friend or a group of friends, play the game first with your friends and have fun with it!

- If you were to be a vegetable, which kind of vegetables would you like to be?

- If you were supposed to wake up as an animal tomorrow morning, which animal would you be?

- If you were to live somewhere on the planet and take all the things you love with you, where would you like to live? What would you take with you?

- What is your favorite color and how this color makes you feel?

- If you were to choose an imaginary friend, who would you choose and why?

- If you were to sit on a bench inside a beautiful forest, who would you like to sit next to you and why?

- Which of these daytimes are you? Dawn? Bright day? Dusk? Or night? Please state why have you chosen these times for yourself?

- If you were supposed to choose an age at which to stay forever, what age would you choose? Why?

- If you were supposed to be in a film, what film would you choose, and which character would you play?

- If you were to meet a historical character, who would you prefer and why?

- If you were to be a city, which city would you choose and why?

- Which 10 foods do you like the best?

- If you were supposed to be a candy, what candy would you like to be? Why?

- If you were supposed to change your name, which name would you choose? Why?

- Which season are you: Spring? Summer? Autumn? Or Winter? Please say why?

- If you get stuck on a remote island, what are the three things you like to be with you?

- Describe your favorite object.

- What is it that you don't have it now but would very much like to have it?

- If you were to choose only one place to spend your vacation, where would you choose and why?

- If you were supposed to say one affirmative sentence for your life, what would it be? (For example: live each day as if it were the last day of your life.)

- Take an important object that is always with you out of your pocket or bag, and tell others why it is important to you?

Once finished, share your answers with your friends and talk about it in your group.

Warm up Games:

It's always better to prepare children's minds and bodies with games designed for such purposes, before starting asanas and other related games. Here, some games are suggested:

- **Walking (Hoohoo, Haha, Hehe, Heyhey)**

Line up the kids and guide them on the walking principles pronouncing a sound when doing the walk, as: walking with the outer edge of the foot (Hoohoo), with the inner edge of the foot (Haha), with the toes (hehe) and with the heels (heyhey). We guide them with these sounds. This game is very suitable for solving the problem of flat feet and knee deviation; it can be played in pairs or in groups of two. Instead of the mentioned sounds, you may also use the sound of different musical instruments or even different musical notes for guiding children. This game will help to increase accuracy, attention and alertness in children.

- **Hop – Nop – Dop – Sop – Lop – Plop**

This game is also a conventional game as we specify a name for each asana. For example: Hop standing straight (Tadasana); Nop: sitting; Dop: bending forward (Uttanasana); Sop: plow (Halasana); Lop: frog (Malasana); Plop: jumping up. Again, children are guided by the teacher's voice; The teacher says one of the words and the children must do it immediately, then the next sound and its related movement. This game greatly considerably helps children to increase concentration and attention power, and also increases children's heart rate, excitement and happiness.

- **Wind and Tree**

Children stand in pairs or in groups. One or more of them become trees (either tree asana or a favorite creative tree), the other or others imitate blowing wind around the trees by blowing with their mouths. The wind blows on them and tries to compromise their balance. This game is used both as a game and an asana practice.

- **Head & Face yoga!**

By showing different feelings through our head & facial and playing with some symbolic gestures, we can move our facial muscles and we're going to call it yoga for our head & face! Let's try some samples and see what you can add into this list:

Yes (Lowering the head)

No (Turning head backward)

Indian yes and no (Right and left chin pendulum movement)

I don't want (Turning head to left)

I don't know (Lifting shoulders)

It's sour (Twisting the face)

My face is long (Pulling the chin down with closed lips)

I am happy (Big smile, showing the teeth)

I am tired (Loosening and hanging face and neck)

I am very upset (Lowering lips and eyebrows)

Yawn (Opening the mouth completely)

I pulled my tooth (Puffing the cheeks and holding them with the palms of the hands showing toothache)

My eyes see the tip of my nose (Squinting the eyes)

Give a kiss! (Puckering the lips, kissing in the air)

My tongue is long!!! (Pulling the tongue out of the mouth and downwards)

I am surprised! (Opening the eyes wide, circling the lips as if pronouncing "O" sound)

I am angry! (Frowning)

I am scared! (Making a scary face, covering the face with hands)

I am disgusted: Pulling the lower lip and chin down

Secret admiration sign: Wink! (Try to wink with both eyes)

I'm pretty: Blinking rapidly

I'm thinking: Turn your eyes to look at the upper corner of the left then right side.

I'm excited: Opening the mouth wide open

I'm peaceful: Sitting in meditation (You can ends the practice by a serene gesture of a face in meditation)

Hold and Hug!

First teach Dog – Cat – Mouse /Cobra – Lion – Mouse asanas. Then ask children to get in pairs, close their eyes and make one of the taught asanas with their bodies. Hearing the bell, they open their eyes; if the asanas of both are the same, they embrace each other, and if they are different asanas, they run after each other. (This game, as well as an ice breaking for students who have already been in their yoga session for a period of time, is also used both as a game and an asana practice).

Earth/Sea/Sky

Let's start like this: The yoga mat is the same as earth or land, outside the mat it is the sea, and jumping toward the ceiling means touching the sky. Now the teacher directs children to be either on the earth, or in the sea or in the sky.

Looking for the Dragon's Tail

In this game, children stand in line. The first student is considered to be the dragon's head and the last one is considered to be the dragon's tail. We set a path. The children start running on this path, the dragon's head (the first child) must try to reach its tail (the last child), and the last child should run away from him by running fast and directing the children in front. The queue should not be separated throughout the game.

Dance of the Joints

In this game, ask the children to walk like a robot or an iron man as if they have no joint; same as a tree trunk! Then the joint can move at any time you touch it. Keep going until all joints are released. Instead of touching, you may use something like a magic wand. They can also play the game in pairs.

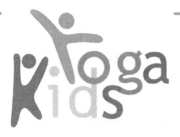

CHAPTER 9
Asanas & Games
Why Asanas (yoga postures)?

Here I introduce you to some traditional yoga postures and some fun moments you can create with the related postures with kids adapted to their age group.

Although all these postures are derived from traditional asanas, I tried to modify them into a form applicable to the children's class. Along with the explanation of each posture, its benefits are also mentioned.

By their nature, children jump and move around most of the time. They do whatever their bodies feel like doing at any given moment. Some of these movements are relaxing and energizing. Asanas help children to find more balance in their movements.

Always check that they're not holding their breath and encourage them to breathe in and out gently, and with a harmonious rhythm.

The most important thing is that the child enjoys being in a posture. If a child is pushing themselves to achieve an asana, they risk injuring themselves and cannot be truly comfortable or happy. Therefore, always encourage children to adjust their body in the posture according to their own limits and to not compare themselves with each other. Even better would be for the teacher to demonstrate the pose with the modifications and tell them that it is perfectly beautiful and ok to be where your body leads you, and that the aim is not to do the pose fully according to what the image of the perfect posture is, but to make the ideal posture for your own body.

Some postures are not recommended for children under the age of eight years old, as their body is still quite fragile. For example, head stands (sirsasana), the complete candle posture or shoulder stand (sarvangasana), the fish (matsyasana), the warriors (virabhadrasana), the deep twist postures (ardha matsyendrasana), and hand balances (ardha mukha vriksasana.)

Always be conscious of the students ages before teaching any asana.

Yoga postures (Asanas) & Some related games

In this section you'll learn how to teach some basic Asanas to kids and enjoy some variations and games along the way.

While reading this section, have in mind that this book is not detailed in the teaching principles of asanas and by using this book it is considered that you already are a yoga teacher who like now to bring the gift of yoga into children's world or you are a practitioner of yoga who have regular yoga practice and already have the knowledge of Asanas or yoga postures and wants to share it with kids.

If some postures seem complicated for you to instruct them to kids please consult an experienced yoga teacher in your city or drop an email to me directly and I'll be happy to come back with any support during your process of learning.

www.nobiehkiani.com

nobieh@nobiehkiani.com

1. Different sitting positions

Items needed: Yoga mat, sitting bolsters & cushions
Most children are usually challenged to sit with a straight back after 8 years of age without any support. It is easy for small children to sit up straight; the older they get the harder it is for them to sit properly with a straight back and opened chest.

In fact, by leaning on comfortable sofas for hours and bending over the desks, we get used to hump. Many yoga sitting games and postures teach children how to sit properly.

First make them sit in a circle. Then ask them to sit straight on the ground in as many different positions as they can. Ask one of them to model and others will follow their friend's position.

Then guide them like this:

"Feel the contact points of your body with the ground. Now imagine that you are rooted in the ground like a plant. How do you feel the ground beneath you? Do you think it is hard or soft? Now move your body a little to left and right, again feel your roots under your body and in the ground, don't you feel more settled now? Now move your body a little to the front. Don't you feel more pressure in front of your body now? Now pull your weight back and lean. Do you feel more pressure in your back? Now change your weight to left and right again; which side do you feel more pressure in? Make your roots tighter on the ground. Now circularly move your body clockwise, and then change to counterclockwise. Slow down the circular movement gradually until it is automatically stopped. Do you think your sitting position has changed now? What change do you feel?"

Ask the children to share their feelings about sitting and its different positions with you and the group then ask them how they felt more comfortable and in which position their back was most straight.

Once explored in different sitting postures, invite them to sit up straight in their favorite sitting position as if they were flowers growing taller toward the sun!

Then ask them to close their eyes for some moments and guide them into some visualization in the sitting posture as follows:

Imagine you are a beautiful flower growing taller toward the sun as you bring your spine nice and straight up, leaning on an imaginary wall, pull your back toward the wall.

Open your chest and have a big inner sunny smile in your heart.

Put a beautiful smile in your lovely face as well!

WOW!

How elegant and beautiful you all look!

Then guide them to breathe properly for a couple of rounds.

then,

Slowly take them back and let them share about their experiences.

NOW,

After they're rooted in their chosen sitting posture, you can guide them into different sitting postures like Padmasana (Lotus), Virasana (Hero), Siddhasana (Perfect pose), Sukhasana (Easy pose), Gomukhasana (Cow Face posture), Ardha padmasana (Half lotus), Dandasana (Staff pose), Svastikasana (Simple Cross-legged), or Baddha konasana (Butterfly pose).

2- Mountain pose (Tadasana)

One of the most important and fundamental principles emphasized in yoga is "the right way to stand". The right way to stand is a position that gives us a feeling of power. In yoga, we usually do this asana barefoot so that we can feel the ground beneath our feet and feel grounded.

"Bare feet are the best shoes for doing yoga asanas!"

Place children along a line with the feet shoulder distance apart from each other, and guide them this way:

"Feel the ground under your feet. Stamp your feet on the ground for a few times. Move your toes. Which parts of your feet are pressed to the ground? Where is your weight centered? Is most of your weight on your heels or under your toes? Try to put an even amount of weight across your whole foot. Make sure each foot has the same amount of weight. You can shift your weight more to the outside of your feet to create an even distribution of weight."

"Feel you are firmly rooted to the ground. Now switch your focus to the other parts of your leg. What do you feel in your ankle, shin, calves, knees, thighs? Unlock your knees and keep them slightly bent."

Stand tall with a straight back. Let your hands hang down to your sides, sending energy to the hands. Keep your shoulders away from the ears and open your chest. Keep your neck long, head high and straight, with the chin tucked in a bit. Imagine you are being pulled up from your head with an invisible string. Now feel like a strong and steady mountain.

You may encourage children to stay in the posture while singing a song:

"As a mountain steady and strong
I'm standing ready and tall
The strongest winds can not make me fall
Let them come cause I'll be ready,

hanging tight and holding steady.
"To the Left, To the Right
To the Front, To the Back" (Repeat 3 times)

When all children reach the "front, back, right and left" part of the song, if they are in a standing circle then they can hold each other's hands and move their bodies in different directions, while their feet are rooted in the ground.

Other ways to do the exercise:

- Instead of moving the whole body to left and right, you may ask them to shift their weights completely on their toes, then heels.

- Ask them to shift their weight completely on to one leg. Move the other leg a little bit and then change sides.

- Instead of singing a song, ask children to get on their heels and toes; therefore increasing their concentration on the movement.

- You may ask them to imagine they are playing a piano with their toes. Together they move their big toe or small toe or all of the toes, and make their favorite key sound; They can play by shifting the big toe while pressing the other toes down and vice versa; or push their own piano keys by their feet while walking, and make a sound with their mouth.

- Another way to make the mountain asana could be a four-person practice, such that three children stand in a circle and hold each other's hands. The fourth child stands in the middle of this small circle, becoming a falling mountain! shifting her weight and falling to the right and left and around the protected circle of 3 friends. The three other children, while holding each other's hands tightly, must make her stable like a mountain with care and support, helping her to not fall and stand still like a mountain. After they help their friend to stand still, they can adjust the posture, like the feet, hands, strait back, relax face, maybe a beautiful smile! :)

Creating a perfect Tadasana in her body, they change their place, and each will have the opportunity to become the mountain.

This exercise is more suitable for smaller children, on a ground covered by a rather soft mat, under your supervision.

3. Tree (Vriksasana)

This exercise improves balance and physical endurance in children. Physical balance has directly a positive impact on mental and emotional balance. It is also very effective in improving their self-confidence and self-reliance. Tree posture is a balance position on one foot, while hands are above the head. First, teach the asana to the children, step by step. Then ask them to spread around the classroom and first begin with mountain posture and then get positioned in tree pose. You may guide them as follows:

"Stand tall, feel the ground under your feet. Without lifting your leg off the ground, put your weight on one side of your body. Wait for a while until you are totally settled in this position. Now, stay strong in the leg you put your weight on and slowly lift your other leg up without losing your balance. The foot on the ground alone holds you. Now lift your free leg from the ground as far as you can, bend it from the knee and put its sole on the inner side of your thigh. When you find your balance, raise your hands slowly and stick your palms together if you can. Remember not to hold your breath during the exercise, and slowly continue your regular breathing. Feel that you are in this position with all your strength. Completely feel your hands which are raised up to the sky and your feet which are rigidly on the ground. When you are ready, return the raised leg to the ground and stand on your both legs again." Repeat the exercise with the other leg, then talk to them about this practice and the feelings they had while doing it.

Other ways to do this exercise:

- If children lose their balance while doing this exercise, you may guide them to better maintain their stability by putting one hand on the wall. Once they are in balance, they can detach their hand from the wall and get into tree position, without the help of the wall. Children between 3 and 5 years old can only put the tip of their toes on the ground. Maintaining balance on one leg is challenging for them.

- While doing balance postures, eyes should not be usually closed, and to better balance, ask the children to find a gaze in front of them and concentrate on that point.

- By counting, you may encourage children to stay more in this posture.

Games related to the tree posture:

- **"Disturbing Wind and the wobbly Tree"**:

One child plays the role of the wind and another one, the role of the tree. By blowing, the branches of the tree move toward the wind, but its roots are firm and stable in the ground. The child tries to keep her balance, and then repeats the tree posture with her other leg. To make it more fun you can ask the child in the tree pose to sing and repeat for 3 times (I'm a wobbly tree…I'm a wobbly Tree…I'm a wobbly tree!) on both sides, before changing roles.

After repeating the game on both legs, the two children exchange their roles and repeat the game.

- **"Naughty snake and the wobbly Tree"**:

Do the same as before; The difference is that the other child plays the role of a snake instead of the wind. She creeps on the ground, twists around the tree and tries to upset the balance of the tree.

-**"Wobbly Tree"** game: Ask children to get into the Tree balance position. Then move their bodies to the left, right, front and back and sing together:

one, two, three! I'm a wobbly tree!

You may also invite children into the circle in turn. The child in the middle goes to the asana, and the rest sing for her and challenge her balance.

-**"Who is Up the Tree?"**:

For playing this game, after teaching the tree asana, ask the children to get in the Tree balance position. Now tell each other in a happy voice: "Who is up the tree?" And then name a creature, for example: "The elephant is up the tree!"

Then, make the Garudasana (eagle pose) hand position with your hands like an elephant trunk. Then without losing balance, move the trunk to left and right. This way, you may invite any animal to the top of the tree, such as: Cow (Gomukhasana or Cow's face pose in hands), Butterfly (winging with hands), Star (hands open to sides), Spy (hands on the eyes like spectacles), etc.

You may even ask the children themselves, and let them use their imagination so that their creativity increases by doing asana and playing at the same time.

-**"Mother fairy may I?"**:

One child is Mother Fairy (you can use other characters like a Superhero or a Guardian depending on your students).

The mother fairy stays on one side of the room with a magical wand in her hand. The other children line up on the opposite wall and imagine they are magical walking trees. Mother Fairy turns away and starts counting. Slowly, the other children start to walk towards her. When she turns towards them, they must turn into a standing tree, and stay balancing for the length of time that she's facing them. If their foot touches the ground and they lose their balance they must go back to the wall and start from the beginning. Play resumes and Mother Fairy turns with her back towards them again and starts counting. Ask them to change legs each time they stand still in tree pose. The one who reaches Mother Fairy first takes the wand and becomes the next Mother Fairy. The game continues as before. Make rules such as 'No running!' and 'No cheating!' Points or praise could be given to those respecting the rules. Emphasize that the aim of the game is to have fun. It's not only about winning. Explain that in yoga games there is no winner and loser. We just play and enjoy!

4-Sun Salutation (Surya namaskar)

Items needed: yoga mat

The sunrise is such a magical phenomena. When darkness disappears and sunshine starts to warm up the planet is a mystical moment...Maybe it's because there is no life on the earth without light. By saying Hello to the Sun in sun salutation, we can express our excitement to this magical moment and breath the sun in our hearts to open our inner smile and start a shiny, magical day.

Sun salutation consists of a series of consecutive and interconnected postures. Actually, it is like a dance consisting of movement and stillness, which can be performed slowly or fast depending on your energy. You should bear in mind that the goal is to do asanas one after the other like a flow.

This series of consecutive postures makes the body strong, flexible and relaxed, while at the same time, amplifies the flow of energy in the body. Deep breathing causes lung cleansing. Natural breathing takes place while doing the postures, so you don't have to draw children's attention to their breathing while doing these postures, unless they hold their breath.

This form of sun salutation which is presented here is designed particularly for children. Children enjoy this series of postures a lot and do them with lots of excitement. While doing these movements, the whole body is invited to move, and after that children become refreshed and cheerful.

Throughout teaching the sun salutation series to smaller kids, you may use the lyrics that are presented in the following, as sample or make your own poems and take them through the series with a song:

"Hello to the Sun"
like a bird's wings My hands are up!
now I tap on the ground with my feet
I bend with my hands on the ground
now I become a mountain, my hips toward the sky
a cat I now become, meow, it is fun
one arm, one leg become flat
the others as well! (other hand and leg)
now I crumple like a mouse
I stand up sharp and smart
I stand,
I spin,
I do whatever I want to…

When doing this exercise, make children sit next to each other, and tell them that you're going to move into different postures like a dance to say Hello to the shiny sun. With the help of a song, you can help children remember the order of movements better. First, repeat the song for a few times, and then show them the movements along with the song. Then ask everyone to stand on their mat and get ready for the flow. Begin the practice in mountain pose, while the palms of the hands are on each other and placed on the middle of the chest as the salutation sign. Begin the practice in a slow rhythm first then by repeating you can gradually move in a faster pace.

Before starting the cycle of movements, ask children to imagine the sun in their minds for a few minutes. Tell them: "Make a shiny image of the sun with closed eyes and feel the rays of the sunshine gently warming your body.

Like a bird's wings, my hands are up.

In standing position, while hands are on both sides of the body, guide the children to slowly move their hands like a circle above their heads, such that they are drawing an imaginary circle around them. This movement causes lateral stretch. Tell them: "With open eyes make a big circle in the space with your hands, look up to the happy, shiny sun and smile to show your appreciation.

Now, I tap on the ground with my feet"

Children, one by one, tap on the ground with their feet; this contact with the ground creates balance and confidence in them. Ask them: "How do you feel the ground under your feet? Is it hard or soft?

I bend with my hands on the ground.

Children will bend forward from the groin area with a straight back and open chest, put their hands on the ground or on their shins (Uttanasana) standing forward bend posture.

now I have become a mountain, hips toward the sky."

Then walk back with their feet, placing their hands on the floor and get positioned as a Down-ward dog (Adho mukha svanasana). Eventually, the body becomes triangular; the hips are pulled upwards like the top of a triangle. This exercise stretches the waist and legs and strengthens the muscles of the arms.

A cat I become, meow, it is fun.

In this position, the child is settled on her two hands and two knees (all fours). Do the cat movement on their back. This cat movement by moving the spine relaxes the back and takes any pressure out of the lower back.

One arm, one leg become flat

The others as well!

After settling in Cat position, now ask the children to straighten their right hand and left leg, and Gaze at a distant point. Repeat this posture with your left hand and right leg.

Now I crumble like a mouse

Ask the children to get in the child's position and try to inspire them with the sense of peace and security. They must feel that they are in a completely calm and relaxed position and are supported by the earth.

I get up sharp and smart

Now they get out of the last position, stand, and look forward with a happy face!

I stand

Then they get into the position of the settled mountain on their feet with a stretched and straight body.

I spin

Spinning is energizing and fun for kids. Ask the children to feel the space around them.

I do whatever I want to…

After spinning, ask the children to move as they like. Remind them that everyone could be in their favorite posture now. Make them understand that being different is a good thing and can add more pleasure to the practice.

You can practice the sun salutation for a few rounds then, ask the children to gather together, and discuss the rhythm and movements. Ask them which movement did they like best and which one did not give them a good feeling, and why? Ask them to demonstrate their favorite posture.

After doing this exercise, guide them to lie on their back and guide them into relaxing their bodies with a few breaths.

Another song for Hello to the Sun exercise:

(in each step guide them into the related posture through the song.

When they got familiar with the postures you can sing the lines then ask them to sing along while going to the posture. You will pose on the particular posture while they will go the the posture when hearing the name of it)

Hold your hands up/ to reach the clouds (Tadasna, mountain pose)
now dive down/back straight and hands on the ground (Uttanasana, Standing forward bend)
put one foot behind/with a soft breath like a line (Chaturanga Asana, plank pose)
give a kiss to the ground/now become a snake on the ground (Ashtanga namaskar, Eight points down pose Then Bhujangasana, Cobra pose)
then the Down-ward Dog/wiggle your tail and make a happy face!
jump forward like a frog/hands to feet, say (ribbit, ribbit, ribbit) (Malasana, squat)
now jump up/see the mountain up high (Tadasana)
Sing:lala lala lalala/lala lala lalala!

Sun salutation Game:

This Game is more adaptable for children above 6 years old.

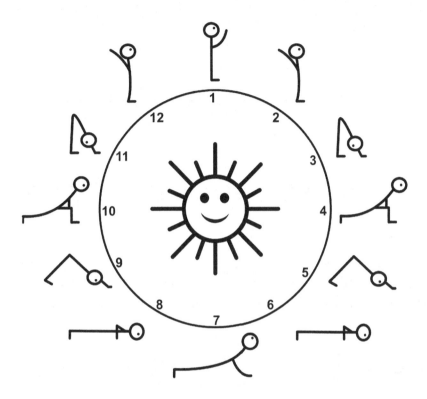

The traditional sun salutation consists of 12 postures.

1- Tadasana (standing posture)
2- Hasta Uttanasana (Raised arms pose)
3- Hasta Padasana (Hand to foot pose)
4- Ashwa Sanchalanasana (Crescent moon pose)
5- Dandasana (plank pose)
6- Ashtanga Namaskara (Eight points pose)
7- Bhujangasana (Cobra pose)
8- Adho Mukha svanasana (downward dog pose)
9- Ashwa Sanchalanasana Crescent moon pose)
10- Uttanasana (Hand to foot pose)
11- Hasta Uttanasana (Raised arms pose)
12- Tadasana (mountain pose)

You may teach the postures with their numbers to the children once; Guide them through it for a few rounds then you can play a game so that they remember the postures and their orders. The game goes as follows:

Gather them in a circle, while one is in the middle of the circle. You will invite the children in the circle to walk in their circle at different speeds guided by one child who is blind folded and stands in the centre of the circle.

The one in the middle who is blindfolded, points her hand to the circle around her, guides the children to circle around in the direction of right or left by repeating a sentence like: go, go, go…Now another side! GO, GO, GO…, and eventually fixes on someone and says: "Stop!"

Then she opens her eyes and chooses a number between 1 to 12 for the child she is pointing to.

The other one should make the posture related to that particular number of the sun salutation series, and the rest repeat the posture after her too. Then she changes her place with the child in the middle and the new child goes on guiding children in the circle. Therefore, this game can keep children concentrated and work on their memory and at the same time they practice their body postures.

5. Frog pose (Squat)

Squatting increases flexibility in the legs.

By jumping like a frog, children strengthen their muscles.

Ask children to squat, open their knees to sides and hold their hips near the ground. Now guide them to put their palms on the ground in front of their rib cage. Ask them to keep their balance by transferring their weight backwards toward the hills and the soles of their feet, imagining that they are happy frogs; Just like a frog, jump up and down and move around the classroom while making its sound. Better for you to also accompany them in the pose to create a sense of trust, also share the enjoyment with them.

Now line up the frogs along an imaginary pond and move to the other side of the classroom while singing the following song. Each frog continues the rest of the way at its own pace while making the sound of a frog.

"Frog Song"

I am a funny frog
I live beside a pond
AND
When the sun starts to shine
I like to jump inside the pond!
Ribbit! Ribbit! Ribbit

You may organize a frog race. All children are lined up at one side of the classroom in the Frog position, and you might use a bell or a whistle then they start moving and jumping to the other side like a frog. How far the race route is or how long it takes depends on the space you have and the creative way you bring more excitement into the game.

6. Mouse pose(Vajrasana) or Rabbit pose (Virasana)

Item needed: yoga mat

In this posture, the child experiences a sense of peace, calm and security. The Mouse posture is also known as the child pose in yoga (Chachangasana), is a good posture to end a yoga sequence of asanas with.

This posture must be done after all back bends; such as Cobra, Swan, Bridge, etc.

First, tell the children to sit on their hills then bend forward to the extent that their foreheads might touch the ground while their big toes are in contact with each other and their knees are slightly apart.

Other ways to do this exercise:

This posture can also be done with open knees. Hands can be placed either on the sides of the body, or on the front and top of the head. While the hands are at the sides of the body, the big toes could be joined together to make a gentle stretch in the sides. knees are wide open, and they will rest their bellies in between the knees.

To make it more fun for kids, This variation of the pose with open knees is called: Rabbit posture (Virasana)

If a kid is challenged to place the hips down to the heels you can place a bolster behind the knees to support the knees then also another bolster or cushion for their head to rest in front of them in case it does not reach the ground.

7- Triangle posture (Trikonasana)

This posture in traditional yoga is called Trikonasana. TRI means three, Kona means corner and Asana means position. Three corners of a triangle.

Can you find the triangles in this position?

Teapot Game:

For smaller children you can use the teapot song as they go into the posture as follows:

Now Let's make the shape of the triangle and become like a teapot!

1- Start from the Mountain pose (Tadasana). Then jump and put your legs 3 shoulders distance apart from each other and the arms are fully extended.

2- Turn your left heel toward the back, pull the toes of the right foot towards the opposite wall and make sure to place the heel of the right foot in a straight line with your mat, right in the middle of the outer edge of the sole of the left foot.

3- Feel strong on the soles of both feet and divide your weight between the two. Relax your toes, put the weight on the outer blade of the left foot under the big toe, heel and the ball of the little toe to feel rooted and strong standing on your feet.

4- Put the left hand on the groin (same as a teapot handle)

5- Bend the right arm in the shape of a teapot spout

6. Now we sing the Teapot song and follow the steps:
   I'm a little teapot
   short and stout
   here is my handle
   here is my spout

7- Now release the left hand from the groin and place it along the leg.
   Straighten the right hand, put it along the right leg and stretch both hand and body.
   When I get all steamed up
   hear me shout:

8- Now bend from the groin to the right side by keeping the rib cage open, and get to the Triangle position.
   "Tip me over
   and pour me out!"
   (Then go to the reverse triangle, imitate drinking your tea!)

9- Now gently get back to the first position, switch arm positions and sing the song again doing the other side.

Tips for instructor to consider:

This posture flexes and strengthens the legs, toes, groin and neck, while it is also very useful for stretching the spinal cord.

Avoid explaining the details of the legs positions to children under 9 as it can become complicated to understand.

For older children who have already practiced for some time, you may explain the details and guide them into the details of the techniques for getting more stable in the posture.

Use of the teapot song for smaller children:

I'm a little teapot
short and stout
here is my handle
here is my spout
When I get all steamed up
hear me shout:
"Tip me over
and pour me out!"

Exercises for older children:

We have three kinds of triangle:

1- Equilateral
2- Isosceles
3- ScaleneAsk the children to create the 3 kinds of triangle in the triangle posture.

8- Butterfly pose (Baddha Konasana)

Ask the children to sit down and bring the soles of their feet together so the soles touch each other, hold the hands on both sides of the feet and open the feet outwards like a book. Ask them to keep their backs straight and stretched and imagine they have a pair of butterfly antennas that allow them to move upward. Now moving your knees up and down, you are colorful butterflies that fly in a garden full of flowers. In such a position, butterflies can fly from one flower to another, while singing a butterfly song you can create with children as the sample below.

In the same sitting position, ask the children to move toward another butterfly, then the next butterfly toward another and so on, until all the butterflies fly once.

Another form of the game:

One of the children is a flying butterfly and the others are motionless. Each of the sitting butterflies may choose the name of a flower, a country or even a color. The flying butterfly chooses one of the children and moves toward her while singing a song. Now it is the next butterfly's turn to move. And this goes on until all the butterflies move once.

Butterfly song:

Look how pretty I am!
See how happy and colorful I am!
What antenas I have! What shiny wings I have!
I like lovely flowers; I like drinking their sweet nectar!
I fly far away, far far away to the magic garden of my favorite flowers!

OR,

The flower sings:

"Butterfly! Where do you go? Butterfly! come to see me soon..."
The butterfly:
"See how beautiful I am!
How happy and colorful I am!
What antennas I have! What amazing wings I have!
I like the flowers; I'm going to sit on them and drink their nectar.
I fly further and further, to the magical garden of colorful flowers!"

- **Cocoon, worm, butterfly, Flower game: (Transformation game)**

One of the games you may play for this asana is the transformation of cocoon to worm, worm to butterfly and ultimately butterfly to a flower on which the butterfly is supposed to sit. In such a way that first we become a cocoon in Virasana position(child pose), then we put the palms on the ground, stretch the head and chest forward, stretch the legs straight from behind, and turn into a worm in the Cobra position (Bhujangasana). Again, we press the palms of our hands to the ground, pull the upper body back, sit, straighten the back, and turn into a butterfly in Baddha Konasana position. Then, in the same sitting position, we place the feed down the ground, bending the knees, seperate the feet hip distance apart, keep the hips open, pass our hands under the knees, With opening the hands wide and open like a big, shiny, beautiful flower!

It's a bit of a balancing posture on the pelvis! So, stay focused and maybe you can name the flower you end up in!

This transformation game can be repeated several times. Flowers may eventually hold the hands of those on both sides in a circle – as the hands pass under their knees – Maybe Sing together a flower song or chant a collective "OM".

*Butterflies Race**: Divide the children to two groups and place them on both sides of the classroom in front of each other. One row settles in butterfly position and the other, in worm position. Worms creep on the ground toward the butterflies. When the worm reaches its opposite butterfly, they change their place, such that the worm becomes a butterfly and the butterfly, in that same sitting position of Baddha Konasana, pulls itself to the other side.

9. Spider pose (Urdhva Dhanurasana)

Items needed: yoga belt, wall

To reach into the complete posture of (Urdhva Dhanurasana), we are going to use the wall and complete the pose as a drop back!

We use the wall to walk downward toward the pose which assembles a walking spider!

Remember to be very mindful in guiding the kids correctly and supporting them confidently in order to protect their lower back and avoid any harms during the process.

To walk them into this posture as explained, you'll need to be a trained yoga teacher yourself or ask someone who knows about the principles of "hand on adjustments" in yoga postures to assist and help you in this posture.

Never take kids into a posture which you don't have knowledge about and haven't had an experience in doing the posture yourself also guiding someone else into it.

Make your sessions safe and free from any danger by getting more confident and first make a priority to get more knowledge and education about anything you want to teach.

Ok, now if only ready to continue. Let's dive into this exciting and refreshing posture!

Invite your students to stand by a wall, one at a time. With the help of a belt, each child bends backwards, bringing their head towards the wall behind them, their hands touching the wall. Slowly guide them to step towards you with their feet, keeping the knees and feet parallel to each other. Then, they can walk their hands down the wall until they touch the ground and arrive in Wheel pose (Urdhva Dhanurasana.) Ask the other children to sing the Spider Song to the child performing the pose to give them energy and support. When the child reaches the ground, let them stay in the pose for a while, then guide them to rest in Child pose until the song has finished. The child can go and play for 2 minutes around the room with other children, then come back and continue with the rest of the group.

> "A spider wise and strong,
> makes his web with love and a smile.
> He's not giving up until he's made it!
> That's how a spider man will make it!
> That super spider you see is me (name of child)!
> I'm happy you could bring your trust in me!
> I am fun and love my friends.

Now tell me would you be my friend? Ok then!

Come and play with me, laughing and jumping and fooling around with me."

You can use the sample songs you have here or come up with your own creative songs and poems.

When the chosen child is walking backward down the wall through his hands in reaching the posture always with your guidance and assistance, invite the other kids to sing along the spider song and encourage their friends to move into the posture.

Other suggested spider songs:

"There's a spider on the wall!
There's a spider on the wall!
If he's careful he won't fall!
He moves slowly DOWN the wall!
I can watch him crawl and crawl!

(When the child reaches the floor, everybody sings to him that rhyme below and invites him to stay in the posture till the end of your 3 repeated songs!):

"There's a spider on the floor!
There's a spider on the floor!
There's a spider on the floor!"

Then slowly take the child out of the posture and continue with another child repeating the same process.

You can choose another version of the song you'll find below and guide them to do the posture by laying on their back then step by step going to the complete pose of Urdhva dhanurasana. You can also create your own spider song and sing along with kids and inspire them to stay in the pose until the song ends.

"A Spider in the web!
A spider in the web!
It can be in many shapes!
Here I see a spider on his web!
Who spin and spin and spin!
He makes a perfect web !"""

10. Chair Posture (Uttkatasana)

Ask the children to stay in Tadasana or Mountain position, ask them to spread their legs shoulder-width apart, and fix the soles of their feet on the ground. Bend their knees a little and lower the pelvis as if they are sitting on a chair, an imaginary chair! Emphasize that they should bend their knees as far as they don't feel pressure on their knees and can see their toes when looking down in that position; that means their knees should not be further than the toes. Abs inside, hips sucked in, so that they can keep their back straight. Keep the chest open such that they are leaning on the back of a chair. Now pull the arms forward and up, and hold the palms facing each other. Look at a point ahead and up and stay in the posture for five inhalations and exhalations. Then straighten their legs, bring down their hands and rest for a few seconds.

Now, Let's try some related and fun games:

Tables Race game:

Divide children into two groups.

One side is all chairs and the other side is all tables (Purvottanasana).

*Go first to the Table pose description coming in the following asanas in this chapter.

For Table posture (Purvottanasana) demonstrate the version in which they have their knees bent so that they can be protected on their lower back and enjoy staying longer in the posture without any unpredicted harm.

The table pose starts with sitting first in a staff pose (dandasan), sitting on your hips with your legs extended and your back straight and strong. Then putting the hands behind with the fingers pointing toward your back. Bending the knees, placing the soles of the feet on the ground, pushing into the hands and feet to lift the pelvic up. bringing the belly button up so that the back is strong and straight as a table.

You can put a yoga block on the belly of each table. When the game starts, the table cautiously moves toward its opposite chair, without letting the block to fall from its belly. If it falls the table will go back and start again from the starting point. When the pair of kids playing along, reach to each other, they change their roles. The other one takes the position of a table and returns to the start point of the race with the block on its belly. The group which reaches the finish line first without dropping the yoga block, wins the game.

This game is recommended for children above 6 years of age.

Elevator game:

After correctly teaching the (Utkatasana) chair pose, ask the children to stand in groups of three. Two children take each other's hands and stand facing each other. The third one stands in between them. In fact, the two children who take each other's hands play the role of an elevator and the third one is the rider. You determine that for example you have 3 floors. The first floor is sitting position, the second floor is Utkatasana (chair position) and the third floor is simple standing. Now the child who is riding the elevator runs the game. She presses the imaginary elevator button and declares which floor she wants to go, 1, 2 and…And stop and hold the position. Each child runs the game between 2 and 3 minutes by continuously guiding the elevator to different floors and then, they change their place.

Other methods to play this game:

- This game can be played collectively. All of them hold hands in a circle and you guide them to different floors.

- You may consider parking, rooftop and…depending on your creativity to make it more fun.

- The number of floors may increase and the chair position on that floor may become heavier or lighter.

Hammock game:

Two children face each other in Utkatasana position, and another one lies down on the ground between them. The two children in that same position grab her hands and feet and swing her gently. Then they change their place.

This game is specifically suitable for older children. In children between 3 and 7 years of age, it is better if two adults (you and your assistant) take turns in swinging the children. In such cases, it is only considered playing and doesn't fall into the category of asanas. Of course, the two children can swing a light weighted doll in Utkata position, which is considered an asana.

The Truck Driver game:

This game is played in pairs. One child settles on the ground in "Happy Baby" pose. The other one settles in Utkatasana with open legs, and takes the feet of the sitting child with both hands, gently pushes her to right and left, and turns the steering wheel as if she is driving a truck; this helps to open the pelvis of the child in the happy baby pose while getting all the other benefits of the chair pose for the child who is on the driver's role. It is also a suiting back massage and lower back pain release for the lying child.

11. Seated Forward bend (Paschimottanasana)

Ask the children to sit in a staff pose (Dandasana), and stretch their legs straight forward.

Now guide them with a funny phrase such: "now point your toes toward yourselves as your toes were saying hello to your face!" Then ask them to raise their hands and bend forward from their hip joints with a strong, straight back and an Open shiny, happy smile in their hearts in order to open their chests, and as you all bend forward in your circle start by moving your toes and say hello to each other by your wiggly toes! "along the way slowly reach for your toes, keeping the shiny smile on your chest…" as they reach down invite them to stay in the posture for a minimum of 3 deep breaths. Then ask them to get back to a simple sitting position and relax their bodies for a while.

Some fun games to explore the posture:

Rocking Chairs game:

Children sit in pairs back to back. One child sits with straight knees in a Dandasana posture, and the other one puts the soles of her feet on the ground and keeps her knees bent. They clasp their hands together up to their elbows. Then, the child with bent knees, pushes her teammate's back and makes her bend forward. This way, her own chest opens and the other child experiences a nice forward bend. If they play the game a few times in a row they will look like rocking chairs!

Cars Race:

The children sit in a Dandasana position, imagining they are seated in a car. To make the game more fun and exciting, first ask everyone the model and color of their cars. Now check the wipers (moving feet right and left from ankle), check the side mirrors (turn to right and left), open and close the trunk (Purvottanasana), open and close the hood to check if the car is safe (Paschimottanasana) and when you get assured that the car is in a good shape, you may guide them to drive their car in the same Dandasana pose for a check, then they will start to drive around always sitted in the same posture. The cars may collide and overturn (Hallasana) and then, the emergency car arrives and puts the car in its initial position.

Play along, use your imagination, and have fun with the game!

Then ask them to lie down, relax and reflect on the posture and the fun they had playing the game.

12. Seated Forward bend with Open Legs (Upavistha Konasana)

You can use a cooking subject to teach this asana. For example, imagine we are going to cook a pizza today. Ask the children to sit together in a big circle with wide open legs. The more open the legs, the bigger the pizza! Like a professional chef, we sit absolutely straight with an Open inner smile (inviting to look confident and open their chests). We keep the knees straight and the toes facing up. We are going to look like a large flat table for spreading the pizza dough. Now, with good care so that our table won't get broken and crooked, we start kneading the dough and spread it well on the table (bending forward and moving hands toward the middle of the circle)

Now that the dough is ready, we may add the ingredients little by little. You may play with variety to the postures here, for example, while you are sitting, turn to the right and take the tomato from your right side. Then turn to the left and take the cheese from that side. reach up and take the salt, reach far to take the pepper…The same way, take the ingredients from around you and put them on the dough, using your own creativity and the children's suggestions and ideas add to the vibrations. You may take different material from the top, bottom, back and…cabinets. In the meanwhile, children are doing the asana and opening the hip joints without getting restless by staying in the posture for a longer time. Finally, by bending forward and putting the pizza on the oven in the middle of the circle you'll complete the posture!

Then you'll stay there (in the forward bend, maybe using your hands under your chin or maybe even lying your head down) and wait for the pizza to be cooked and ready to eat!

Variety of the game:

- Instead of pizza, you may bake a cake or bread or anything else you might come up with your own creativity. At the end of the class, you may even surprise the kids with the real food you have already prepared ahead so that you can share it with them at the end of your session, in case they get hungry due to the subject!

13. Table posture (Purvottanasana)

Ask the children to sit on the floor, put the soles of their feet on the ground in front of their bodies, and bend the knees. Now put their palms on the ground behind their pelvis the way the fingers are facing forward. Keep the rib cage totally open, lift the pelvis up from the ground. Tell them: "Make your stomach flat like a table and pull your pelvis as high as you can. I want to put a few vases on these flat tables! Let me see if you can be so flat & stable that the vases don't tilt and fall."

After staying in this posture for a few breaths, ask them to gently put their pelvis on the ground, hug their knees to their chest and rest for a while.

For children above 8 years old, you can use the more advanced version in which the legs are stretched forward instead of bending the knees.

Some fun games with the asana:

- One game you already explored was in the section you learn about the chair posture (Utkatasana). Go back to the related Asana and enjoy playing the game one more time.

- Tell them you are supposed to turn into a crab near the sea. Make the Table asana and walk to the right and left like a crab.

-Tables or Crabs race:

Place them in separate groups in pairs. One member of each pair settles on the opposite side of the class in table position (Purvottanasana). Put a yoga block on the stomachs of those who made the Table asana and ask the tables to hold the blocks so carefully that they don't fall off their bellies. With the guidance and encouragement of the groups in front of them, they will move forward in the same pose toward their partner in game, if the block falls they will go back and start from the beginning point. Any table who carries the block to the other side of the classroom while keeping the block on its belly, hands over the block to its partner and the other child will go back to the other side respecting the same rules. The pair who walked slowly, carefully and carried the block to each other with respecting all the game's rules wins!

14. The Downward dog posture (Adho Mukha Svanasana)

You can use many creative ideas to get the kids to perform this pose. For example, you can ask kids to visualize a mountain and make the shape of a high mountain with the body:

"Children, do you know what the peak of a high mountain looks like?"

Children do this posture naturally from a very young age and enjoy playing with it in their yoga games.

Guide them to go to all fours in cat posture (marjaryasana). Placing the palms of the hands on the ground, tucking their toes under, getting stable in this posture then, first Let them move their bodies a little in the cat pose, making waves in their spine, opening their mouths and if the group age you are working with are under 5 making the sound of a cat: miauuuuuuuuuuuuuuu!

Then ask them to get still in the posture and start by separating their knees from the ground and lifting their buts up and try to bring the sole of the feet near to the ground.

Now they are in the downward dog!

You can ask them to stay in the posture and play with your funny ideas you'll guide them into:

- Make waves in their spine.

- Wiggle their tails!

- Lift their legs up one by one and look like a dog who goes for a pee!

- They can bounce on their feets like an excited dog!

Then Freeze in the posture for 3-5 deep breath...

And ask them to go to the mouse pose (child pose) to rest.

Variety of games for dog posture:

-Horse and Carriage game:

In this game we will use 3 postures:

1- Downward Dog (Adhomakha svanasana)
2- chair pose (Utkatasana)
3- Stretching in a backbend

Divide the children to groups of three. In each group, one child is the carriage driver (Utkatasana), one child is the carriage (Downward Dog) and one child is the horse (Backbend).

First the one on the downward dog will be the carriage and is the first one getting ready in the posture.

Then the horse is getting ready by your step by step guidance into the posture:

1- Place your feet hip distance apart facing the spine of the child in downward dog
2- Place your hips on the lower back part of the spine of our downward dog
3- Slowly start to bend backward, putting her spine in line with the spine of our downward dog
4- Stretch your hands over your head.

Now,

We have our third group member already being ready on the other side on our downward dog and she will get into a chair pose by bending her knees and with a straight spine, holding the hands of the second child who is playing our horse in a backbend.

As you can see, we have a carriage with a horse and a driver!

Change roles so that each child will do all 3 postures.

-Tree/Bridge/Stone:

Gather kids in groups of 4.

We will have 3 asanas.

1- Downward dog (Adho Mukha svanasana): Here represent our bridge
2- Tree posture (Vriksasana): The tree
3- Mouse posture (virasana/child pose): Here represent our rock

3 kids will each go to one of those postures and stay in the pose.

The fourth child will start by:

Going around the tree,
passes under the bridge,
jump over the rock,

then he becomes a tree and the tree will come out of the pose and be the one going through the steps.

The game will go on until everybody has a go in each role.

Additional Notes:

- For more advanced classes and children above 6 you can use (Urdhva Dhanurasana) the wheel posture for the bridge instead of the downward dog pose, or you can even add this posture as a second bigger bridge and use 4 asanas for kids to explore.

- Remember that each time you want to introduce these games you first need to instruct the asanas one by one, let them explore the postures then take them into the game.

15. Plank posture (Chaturanga Asana)

This posture is suitable for children above 6 years of age. Smaller children may not be strong enough to stay in this pose and get tired soon because they still don't have enough developed muscle in their hands and back to stay in this posture.

Ask the children to get on all fours. Place their hands firmly on the ground and straighten their elbows without overstretching it. To avoid the over stretching in the arms, you can guide them to slightly micro bend their elbows and place their arms in a way that their inner elbows will be parallel to each other. Now stretch their legs backwards one by one, tucking the toes under, straighten their knees and push their heels back. Straighten their body in one line, like a plank.

Remind them to be straight and strong looking like a heavy plank and not a soft, fragile, and broken plank! The important point in this asana is that the back isn't curved, and the head isn't hung. After 3 to 5 breaths, take them into child pose for the back muscles to rest for a while.

Variety of games to explore in plank asana:

- You may refer to the "Creative games "section on this book and use Crocodile games, and select one of those types of games, which is created with the same asana.

- Side plank (vasisthasana): when the children have mastered the plank posture, you may take them to this position, and ask them to gradually put their weight to one side of their body, for example to the right. Now ask them to remove their left hand from the ground, turn the body to the right and at the same time, remove the left foot from the ground, then put it on their right foot in pairs or a little higher. They can stay in this position for 3 breaths, and then shift sides.

- Gate: they can settle in the "side plank" position. If we move the upper and the pelvis up and down at the same time, it looks exactly like opening a gate. You can use this form as the main gate of the city to design a class like a tour in the city and...

16. Creating a vinyasa cycle

Vinyasa means coordinating the asanas & breath in a flowing cycle.

Moving into the asanas one after the other. This method of yoga is called Vinyasa flow.

In Vinyasa flow asanas flow one after another like a dance.

For making a Vinyasa cycle, asanas should be taught separately in former sessions. The asanas used in one cycle should be interchangeable and interconnected.

You can use stories and some creative themes taking the kids into a journey while they are creating the vinyasa cycle with your guidance.

Remember it is important to mention the key points of each asana while performing the cycle.

Make it simple, easy to understand, fun and create a story which awoke their curiosity to follow your story and bring excitement to wait for the next posture to turn into.

Choose asanas which can easily follow one after another.

Let's start with some simple samples.

Follow the steps below to make a sample Vinyana cycle:

Sample 1

Postures in order:

1. Cat (Marjariasana)
2. Downward Dog (AdhoMukha Svanasana)
3. Upward Dog (Urdhva Mukha Svanasana)
4. Rabbit (Virasana or child pose)
5. Cobra (Bhujangasana)
6- Mouse (Vajrasana)

- First we get into all fours (the arms and legs are shoulder-width apart). With a deep breath, we lift the head and tailbone, and by exhaling, we bend the back inwards; pulling the head and tailbone inwards (like a cat who is relieving fatigue in its back).

- Then while the weight is under the ball of the toes, we pull the hips up and the rib cage inward (Down-he Dog).

- Now we pull the body up, and open the rib cage (Upward Dog), while the shoulders are pulled backwards and far from the ears.

- Then we pull the hips toward the heels, and bring the rib cage closer to the ground (Rabbit)

- With a deep breath, we press the palms on the ground, bring the upper body forward, place it on the ground from below the navel, slightly bend back the elbows and settle in Cobra position.

- Then, we pull the hips toward the heels, bring the knees close together and place the hands next to the body while they are completely relaxed (Mouse).

Sample 2:

1. Mountain position (Tadasana)
2. Standing Side bent (Tiryaka tadasana)
3. Standing Forward Bend (Uttanasana)
4. Hand eagle pose (Garudasana)
5. Downward Dog (Adho Mukha Svanasana)
6. Lion's Breath (Simhasana)
7. Frog (Malasana)
8. Plank (Chaturanga Asana)
9. Salut Eight Points of Body (Ashtanga namaskara)
10. Cobra (Bhujangasana)
11- Mouse position (Virasana)

And we begin the cycle like this:

"First we stand firm, straight and high like a mountain (Tadasana), to look around, slide to right and left (Tiryaka Tadasana), bend down from your hip joints (Uttanasana), we have an elephant who comes to the pond, playing with water with its trunk (hand Garudasana), moves its trunk to right, left, up and down, bringing its head down, it sees a dog (Adho Mukha Svanasana),

We have a very excited dog!; it stretches his body forward (Urdva muka svanasana) and laughs (Lion's Breathing),

The dog suddenly sees a frog (Malasana or a squat). The frog starts jumping, up & down, then jumps back into a plank!

Then the knees and chest comes down, elbows bend, it comes down and kisses the ground (Salut Eight Points of Body),

Suddenly a snake emerges from behind a rock (Bhujangasana or Cobra) and begins to make a "hissssssssssss" sound. Once the small mouse sees the snake and hears its voice, cuddles and hides (mouse pose or Virasana).

Sample 3:

The asanas to be used:

1- Cat (Marjariasana)
2- Tiger(Bidalasana)
3- Downward Dog (Adho mukha svanasana)
4- Upward Dog(Urdhva Mukha svanasana)
5- Downward Three Legged Dog (Tri pada adho mukha svanasana)
6- Boat posture (Navasana)
7- Sitting twist (Marichiasana)
8- Sitting Bent Forward(Paschimottanasana)
9- Dog post (Adho Mukha svanasana)
10- Cat pose (Marjariasana)
11- Mouse pose(Vajrasana) or Rabbit (Virasana).

The story to create this Vinyasa cycle:

We have a cat (Marjariasana) in our house,

Sometimes she thinks that she is a tiger, and (Bidalasana) shows its paws and sharpens its tail like a tiger! Right hand, left leg stretches and changes sides.

We also have a dog (Adhomukhasavanasana) which is very cute,

both of them when get tired and yawn are so cute (urdhva mukha svanasana),

we have to take our dog out for a walk twice a day. It constantly jumps here and there, pees and sets signs not to get lost (Tri pada adho mukha svanasana), Lifting the legs up one by one in downward dog.

One day I went to the riverside along with my lovely dog and cute cat, then we had to get back home with a boat (Navasana).

We were tired so we started to twist our bodies into the left and right (Marichiasana)

We then reached home and slowly disembarked (Paschimottanasana),

The dog jumped out!(Adho Mukha svanasana)

Then the cat! (Marjariasana),

And finally we all took a rest together, mouse or rabbit pose (Virasana or vajrasana)

Variations of this exercise

1- Ask a child to perform an asana. The next child should copy the first asana and add another pose to it. They should continue until every child has added a different posture to the cycle, creating a vinyasa cycle.
Divide the children into two groups with each group creating its own vinyasa cycle. Both groups can then show their cycle to the other group.
2- Create a vinyasa flow cycle by telling a story including yoga postures in it. As the children listen to the story, they can move into the relevant poses.
3- Alternatively, start the story and then ask each child to add to the story, and add an asana as well, creating a group story and vinyasa cycle.

Some more variations you might add to make it more fun!

*Ask the children to imitate the sound of the animal related to each movement.

*Ask each child to perform an asana; the second child should first do the previous asana and then their selected asana, and so on. Each child adds a posture to the cycle, and this way, the children make their own Vinyasa cycle.

*We can divide children into two groups. Each group makes a Vinyasana cycle as mentioned above; then each group performs its cycle for the other group.

*Practice and design a Vinyasana cycle by using 10 chosen asanas; then you can also add a story on it and practice playing with combining the story which goes along into the vinyasa cycle. Make sure your story is not too long and is interesting enough to create a sense of curiosity and excitement for kids to play along with you. Also choreograph the cycle in a way that asanas easily flow one after another and it's easy and logical for the body to move from one asana into another.

Teaching different Asanas:

You may teach different yoga asanas according to children's age and class status. For children between 3 and 5 years of age, as described at the beginning of this book, you may use different animals with images, related games, or your creative illustrations. Remember to never correct children at this age, don't use reverse postures, heavy back bends and Warrior postures.

For children between 5 and 8, you may use a variety of asanas. In each yoga session, teach one of the yoga poses; Then use one of the games related to that asana or combinations of few asanas as we went through in the asana samples we already explored in the last chapter.

To children between 8 and 11 year of age, you should teach asanas more accurately and use correct techniques. In this age group, you may teach a few relevant asanas in each session and take your time to explore the mentioned games. Always consider the age of children and the correct use of the practices and games appropriate for their age and condition. For teaching asanas to children, try to choose asanas that you have mastered completely yourself and have experienced in it, know the complete posture if you want to teach more advanced asanas and how it feels in your own body, so that you can correctly convey them to children; with demonstrating the asana correctly yourself you can encourage the children to do the same. They will always mirror you and you are their example so your regular practice is very essential for your teaching.

Ask them to go to the posture within their strength and bodily limitations, find the best position in their bodies and sufficiently and use modifications if needed. Children's bodies are soft and flexible, but the fact that children are able to easily perform many asanas doesn't mean that the posture is necessarily suitable for their young bodies; you should always keep this in mind and choose asanas adapted to their group age and body capabilities. Limiting your teaching is necessary in taking them into some of the yoga asanas (as mentioned earlier in the first chapter), binding you to design your class on the basis of the children's age group and conditions, thus making a beneficial, safe and happy class which is pleasant and useful for them.

Here, You'll be introduced to some fun games and themes you can use in your classes in order to create an exciting, unique and exceptional yoga session.

ASANAS & Some more fun GAMES

Asana and freeze:

Play a music preferably with the sound of nature and jungle then ask the kids to start by imitating an animal and move around the class playing the role of that animal. When the music stops, each child freezes in their own animal state, then they guess each other's animal in the frozen posture.

Any child who's animal pose has been guessed can come out of the posture and play along by guessing the others posture. Once they all came out of their posture, you can continue in another round by playing the music again. This game improves children's creativity and use of imagination, also they get to know about different animals.

Yoga, yoga, yoga, Asana:

Children sit in a circle. One of them walks around the circle with a magical wand (you can use a feather, a magic stick, a big and funny straw or anything fun which can relate to your class theme).

The chosen child going around the circle gently touches everyone with the magic stick in her hand, while saying the word "Yoga" then after a couple of repeated "yoga" she stops on one child and says "Asana" instead of "Yoga". The child who's been touched by the stick and heard Asana goes into her chosen asana and starts by running after the child having the magic stick in her hand keeping the posture she chose. The child with the stick runs until she reaches the primary seat of the child who is now running after her and takes her place.

Then they will start another round with the new child having the magic wand.

Try to continue until at least all of them once had the magic stick.

A trip to India:

You can dedicate a class session to a trip. Here is an example of a trip to India.

In some sessions you can collect some information about a particular place and prepare some files in the form of movies, illustrated pictures, photos...and take them into a journey in a specific place in the universe. Maybe a country as our example here to India. Or to the moon, to the desert, under the sea...Use your imagination and plan a creative, exciting session in which children will go into an imaginary place, travel with them into an adventurous destination. They will be invited to move their bodies into different yoga asanas while you bring lots of fun as well as useful tips and insights about different subjects related to our universe, all inside your exceptional yoga session.

When they leave, they will feel as if they came out of a magic land full of adventure and can't wait for their next journey in the yoga land!

Now, Let's travel together to the mystical, colorful and amazing country called INDIA!

Sitting in a circle, you may first ask kids to sit in the Butterfly position (Baddha Konasana) and open the soles of your feet away from each other, like an opened book. Look into the book for some information about your trip. (Remember that during your guidance in the story, you should not get lost into your story and forget to mention the important points of each asana, for example Opening their chest, keeping the shoulders away from their ears, breath properly, keeping the back straight...)

Then, in the same position, you can lift one foot with your hands, get it close to your ears and open the hip joint, as if you are speaking on the phone to book your tickets for the trip. They will change legs to make other calls, like calling their friends to invite them to come along and you'll change legs up to 3 times calls with both legs! In between calls you can have both legs up when the line gets busy and you put one on the caller id!

Once explored some sitting postures adding on to your planned story, they will stand up and get ready to take the road toward the airport!

You can ask them to go to Warrior 3 posture (Virabhadrasana 3), get on the plane and go to India. You may then take a bus for sightseeing in the town, such that one who has a stronger body leans to the wall in the Chair posture (Utkatasana) and the others take turns in making the Chair position in front of the previous one with sitting gently on his thighs. All of them form a 2-person or 3-person bus-like queue, and slightly bend to right and left under the guidance of the instructor, you can create a fun environment by imagining a bumpy road or the driver suddenly braking and they will all lean forward!

After the bus ride, they reach The Ganges lake. There, they meet the turtles (Kurmasana).

They get in the boats (Navasana), the cows are walking slowly around it (Gomukhasana), the elephants are taking a bath (you can guide them in Malasana(squat) or Uttanasana (standing bending forward) take your hands in Garudasana in front of your face as the elephant's trunk, and take the elephant for a shower!).

They then get on the train (one after another they sit on the ground in Upavistha Konasana and put their hands on each other's shoulders. You'll be the driver and guide them to move to right and left, back and forth) as a train moves.

Again use your energy and creativity to make the journey more exciting and fun by adding train sounds, stops, bumps...The train can even turn into a spaceship and they will enjoy using their imagination to travel into a fantasy world you will create for them.

Once arrived you'll take them to visit the monkeys (Hanumanasana), snakes (Bhujangasana), pigeons (Eka pada rajakapotasana) and Bengal tigers (Bidalasana). Take them to Taj Mahal (you may stand in the circle and do the Chair pose (Uttakatasana) To assemble the Taj mahal monument). Then, enter the temple and sit in (Lotus), lie on your back and invite them to the ending posture (Savasana) by playing soft classical Indian music and reviewing the memories of the trip.

Remember that you can use the Train game, Bus game, etc. in other games you design.

Needle and Thread:

This is the same jump back and forth during a Vinyasa cycle. We are in the Downward Dog pose. Gaze in between your hands and bend your knees, bounce a few times on your feet then jump through, without moving your hands, crossing your legs and sitting in between your hands. This jump through in between hands looks like a thread passing through the needle hole!

We follow the same principals to jump back! Starting with crossed legs, hands on both sides of the hips. Without moving the hands, move your legs and jump back into a plank!

Relax in child pose for a couple of breaths.

Snake and charmer:

Two children play along; one plays the role of a cobra and the other plays the role of a charmer.

The Cobra starts in mouse posture (Vajrasana) assembling a cobra sleeping in his basket!

The charmer plays his flute and The snake slowly wakes up and comes out of the basket, where the child will go to (Bhujangasana) cobra pose.

The charmer plays his flute and the snake follows the sound…

They can have fun by the charmer moving around the cobra and the cobra will dance along the charmer's flute always staying in the posture!

Ultimately the charmer puts the cobra back in the basket (Virasana/mouse).

Gently massages the back of his friend, like rocking the basket to calm the cobra to sleep again.

Surfing:

We imagine that the yoga mats are surfing boards and we are surfers.

First we lie on our stomach on the mat, lift our chest and move our arms as if we were moving the board toward the waves (Shalabhasana). Then we wait for the wave to come; we find our balance, stand on the board (mat) as if we were standing on the surfing board. Here they can go to warrior 2 posture (Virabhadrasana 2) move our bodies to right and left as if we are floating on the waves, exploring both sides on the postures by changing legs.

You can play with the posture by reversing the (virabhadrasana 2), By bending the knees and going to the side angle (Parsvakonasana) and enjoy the imaginary surfing!

Then go to a child pose to relax.

Tunnel Games:

Children just love to pass under tunnels and bridges!

You can use the idea of making a tunnel with the children in many different games and themes.

To create tunnels, you can use the following postures:

Urdhva Dhanurasana (wheel), Prasarita Padottanasana (wide legged forward bend), vasisthasana (Side plank), Setubandhasana (Bridge), Adho Mukha Svanasana(Downward dog), Purvottanasana (upward plank pose/ Table pose), Marjariasana(cat).

It is such that one child makes the given asana, the next one passes under her body and makes the same asana beside her. The third one passes under the body of the previous two and again makes the same asana beside them, so they continue the tunnel like this. When the tunnel is complete, now the children get out of the asana one by one, pass through the tunnel and settle next to each other in the Mouse position to take a rest.

Note that you should use the more advanced asanas like Urdhva Dhanurasana, vasisthasana... for older children. Also select the number and timing of the asanas so that staying in the postures is not beyond the children's ability.

Colored Balls Factory:

Items needed: small colorful foam balls, baskets or bags for the number of divided groups

In this game, three asanas are used:

1- Virabhadrasana 2(warrior 2).
2- Paschimottanasana (seated forward bend)
3- Shalabhasana (locust pose) and

We divide the children into groups of three.

We are supposed to have a ball painting factory.

We have some small balls for each group with the same number. let's say 6 balls each group of 3.

We put the empty basket next to the first child who is going to do the warrior 2, posture.

Also, the 6 small balls are next to the first player.

She'll be placed at the beginning of the line we will make with the 3 players, and she'll go to the posture.

Next one is sitting in Dandasana posture having her back to the warrior. She'll go from Dandasana to Paschimottanasana once the game begins.

The third child will lie on her belly feet to feet from the second player. She'll go to shalabhasana once the game begins.

Now that we have all in their position, let's go through the game:

The warrior takes a ball, bending from her hip joint facing the back of the second player. She handed over the ball to the second player now in dandasana.

The seated child has the ball in between her 2 hands, bends forward and places the ball in between the ankle of our third player who, now receiving the ball, goes to shalabhasana, raising her legs and hands at the same time for 3 times, assembling painting the ball in a color!

After 3 times, up & down from our Locust, means the ball is painted!

Then we reverse the procedure!

The seated child goes back again to paschimottanasana, collects the ball from the Locust, She takes the ball up above her head and with a gentle backbend hands it over again to the first player, our warrior. She now has the ball in one hand, she reverses the legs and goes to the other side of the posture and puts the ball also in the opposite hand.

Then she places the ball in the basket next to her.

We'll put a timer, let's say 15-20 min to play the game.

Then, the instructor will ring a bell to announce the ending of the game.

We'll count every group's basket to see how many balls each group could collect playing along the game.

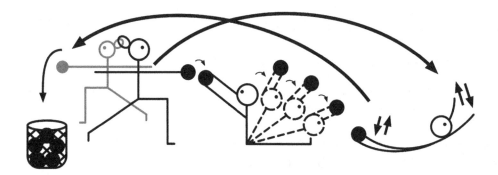

Note for the instructor:

During the game remind them of the important teaching points in each asana. For example: open your chest, bend from your hip joints, stretch your arms, open your chest, happy smile on your face...

Sun Bath game:

This is another partner game. You can use this partner pose in one your beach team, or anywhere they can visualize sunbathing!

In this game, one child settles in the Mouse posture (Vajrasana) or Rabbit (Virasana), playing the role of a sunbed.

The other one is the person sunbathing. She will place her bottom at the end of the spine of her friend in mouse posture. Then she will lie back, opening her chest in a backbend.

In this posture the one in the mouse will receive a nice massage on her back and the one on top will benefit from an open chest and a nice stretch on her back.

Mother and baby asana:

An interesting idea to use other variations in some asanas is to play Mother and baby; in such a way that you first introduce an asana then you ask kids how the baby version would look! Then you demonstrate a variation of the posture and kids will go to both the mother and baby version of the pose.

Here some samples are named:

Cobra:

Mother-----------> Bhujangasana
Baby---------------> Cobra with bent knee
Flamingo:
Mother-----------> Balance posture on one foot and the hand in place of the beak
Baby---------------> The same posture with kneeling.
Dolphin:
Mother-----------> Dolphin pose (Bending the elbows and placing the elbows down on downward dog)
Baby---------------> The same posture in cat posture, with the knees on the ground.
Giraffe:
Mother-----------> Standing tall. palms together and stretched up and high
Baby---------------> The same posture while kneeling
Crow:
Mother-----------> Bakasana posture
Baby---------------> The same movement on forearms
Elephant:
Mother-----------> Standing, hands in Eagle position assembling the elephant's trunk
Baby---------------> The same posture in seated pose.
Tree:
Mother-----------> Vrikshasana
Baby---------------> The same while kneeling
Downward Dog:
Mother-----------> Adomukhashvanasana
Baby---------------> The same posture while kneeling down
Rainbow:
Mother-----------> Side plank (Vasisthasana)
Baby---------------> The same posture with the hip on the ground

Moon:

Mother----------> Ardha Chandrasana posture (half-moon posture)

Baby--------------> The same posture while having the knees on the ground

Eagle:

Mother----------> Garudasana

Baby--------------> The same posture seated

Cat:

Mother----------> Marjariasana

Baby--------------> The same movement on the forearm

And ultimately, you may introduce a hip opening posture which looks like holding a baby and embracing it!

Find a seated posture, lift one leg up and hold it in your arms as if you were holding a baby!

Then by going to left and right while hugging your baby which is your leg you hugged! You are now working on opening your hips and hip joints.

Tell them to kiss their babies by lifting the leg higher and kissing their knee!

You can remind them to be a happy mother by lifting their chest up and straightening their backs.

Then you can tell them they are twins and change sides!

Finally,

You can end your mother and baby session in a posture called: HAPPY BABY!

In which you lie on your back, hold the outer side on your feet with your hands, open the hips and rock to left and right, while pushing your knees down!

You really look like a happy baby! don't you?!

Just look at babies and find them do this posture constantly!

Asana base game:

This game is played by your verbal guidance like a riddle. The children stand in a circle. Guide them this way: "Show me an asana in which your two hands and one leg are considered your pile!" Based on the asanas they have been taught so far, they should find an asana in which they have both hands down the earth and one stands on one leg, so they have 3 bases to make them stable in the pose. They might come to (Tri Pada adho mukha svanasana), lifting one leg up in downward dog pose.

In the same way, you tell them what their pillars will be and ask them to come up with their thoughts and do their guessed poses;

Here are some more examples:

One hand and one foot------> Bidalasana (In cat posture lifting and stretching one hand and the opposite leg)

hips------> Navasana (Boat posture)

Two hands--------> Bakasana (Crow pose) and its variations, balancing on 2 hands.
One foot----------> Any standing balance postures such as (Vriksasana (Tree), Natarajasana(Dancer), virabhadrasana 3 (warrior 3),...)

Sculptor & The Stone:

This is a partner game. One has the role of a stone and settles in the Mouse posture or Virasana on the ground. The next one is a sculptor who wants to carve a beautiful art out of the big stone!

The game should be played in silence and you can play smooth, classical music to invoke the sense of creativity in the sculptor.

The sculptor first looks at the big stone and thinks about his craft.

Then start by making his craft.

He will move the stone in different shapes, the stone just follows the touches she receives from the sculptor.

The sculptor finally will turn the stone into a shape, which will be suggested to be a yoga posture.

Then you'll ask the stones who now turned into some art craft by their sculptor to stay and freeze in the pose, and ask all the sculptors to go around and observe other sculptures as if they were in an art exhibition!

They can take imaginary pictures and admire the arts!

Then, ask them to change roles.

Animal mix machine:

For this game we're having an imaginary machine we call: Animal mix machine!

It looks like a washing machine.

Children will sit in a circle and you're going to call on 2 asanas one by one. The kids will go to the posture.

Let's say for an example: lion & giraffe.

After going to the lion posture, then the giraffe (standing tall, bringing both hand up above the head while having the palms joined together),

Now,

You're going to tell them that it's time to go to the Animal mix machine!

You'll ask them to close their eyes, hug themselves and turn fast to the right & left, while whispering a sound as if a machine is turning....

Then meanwhile you'll ask them to think about and imagine what the new creature which is a mix of lion and giraffe will look like?

Then once you announce to turn off the machines, you ask them to open their eyes & the new mixed animal will come out the machine!

Maybe it's standing tall with a lion face!

Maybe it's sitting like a lion with the long neck and head of a giraffe by bringing the hands up their heads!

Play along in a few rounds, choosing different animals.

This game is fun, inviting kids to learn the postures, use their bodies & imagination to create new movements, also inviting them to silence by engaging their mind & body.

Police asana game:

One child stands in the middle of the circle and goes to a yoga posture, But in a wrong way!

Now the rest of the children who are standing around in a circle, whistle as a police officer, go toward her one by one and each of them corrects one fault in the way he is situated in the posture.

They will go one by one and adjust a movement which corrects the body in the right way it is supposed to be in the asana.

This game helps children to learn more about a correct way of going to a posture, and makes them alert about the adjustment they can do once they are going to the corrected posture themselves.

Variety of the game:

- This game can be played in pairs as well.

- Everyone will go into a yoga posture, one child plays the role of the police. She'll go around and find what's wrong and what can be adjusted then she can put a sticker on the part which needs to be corrected so that the chief police (you) finds the stickers and corrects the pose. You'll go to the next round once everyone has been corrected. The next police is the one with less stickers!

Yoga riddle game:

This Game is very interesting and entertaining at the same time very informative. Children will accompany you with enthusiasm.

In this game, you start the game by revealing some information about a chosen asana. For example, if you consider Cobra (Bujanghasana), you can reveal some information about the snake as a riddle and let children guess what the posture is about and once they find about it then they'll go to the posture. The riddle can be in the form of speaking as the chosen animal or item related to the asana. For the cobra you can say: "I'd like to say hiss…I creep on my belly and have no hands and feet. What am I?"

One fun way to propose the game is to prepare or get some cards. In one part you can have the picture of an animal or any other subjects you choose for your class, on the other side of the cards you'll have some interesting information about the subject.

Kids can choose a random card, or you can put a card under each kids yoga mat. Then they will one by one secretly look at their card, then read some pointed infos about the subject.

The others will guess what it is and go to the related posture.

This game will help improve children's (or even your) general information about animals, plants, flowers, any other species you will introduce to your class.

Suggested PRACTICE:

Design 5 riddles for each age group. The answer to the riddles could be any of the asanas. Design the riddles for different age groups of 3-5 years old/6-9 & 9-12.

Practice to Evoke your own creativity:

As mentioned before, creativity of the instructor is of the most important key points in children's yoga sessions. To increase and cultivate your creativity, It is a good thing to practice on designing and executing yoga games.

Now that we've been through some fun and amazing ideas together let's enhance this inspiration and evoke more of your own creativity.

One of the most enjoyable times I had in the process of working with kids was to get ideas and inspirations from different sources to come up with fun games to introduce into my children's classes.

I'm sure you'll also enjoy this process.

Let your inner child play and have fun. I can guarantee that if you really Enjoy playing these games, trust your intuition and come up with your own creative ideas, you and the kids will have an unforgettable yoga time together!

Here a suggested practice in this regard is presented:

Select 3 asanas and design a game with them. Then first play this game with your own friends. Consider all details while playing the game; the security level of children, the goals of the game, the correct use of asanas in the game, the message of the game, etc.

In addition to practicing playing the game with your friends, it also helps to nurture your inner child and I'm sure your friends also will enjoy it a lot. Remember that if you have fun playing and introducing your games to your class, kids will follow, and they will also enjoy it.

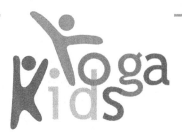

CHAPTER 10
Asanas and Their Benefits

In this section, in order to increase the instructor's information about the effects of the postures or asanas, the benefits of some asanas are briefly mentioned.

Before I go to the list, let's talk about the "Advanced postures and their benefits".

They are mentioned here from number 31 (Head stand).

In this Training book, teaching of Advanced postures is not included. While conducting yoga kids ttc training, I go through all the details of teaching these asanas correctly and with lots of care and modifications.

If you like to know more, you need to learn the proper postures from an experienced yoga teacher in your area.

Remember that always be mindful and teach something you totally know how to handle and introduce it in a proper and safe way. By this you'll avoid any accident or harm during your sessions.

Importance and Benefits of Advanced Asanas and Reversed Postures

Over time and by children's mastery of the instructed asanas, they gradually feel the need for experiencing more advanced postures.

If the instructors decide to teach such asanas to children, they should first work on themselves in order to confront their body, their fears and their challenges. So always try to teach something that you master, and make sure you guide the children correctly. Remember that in doing such asanas, it is as important to cultivate a sense of courage and self-confidence as to be cautious and watchful. So be a guide who, in addition to knowing the child's body and ability, knows the asana well and doesn't make the child scared. The advantages of reverse postures include independence; since we human beings are used to always walk on our feet, practicing standing on the head and hands is unusual then bring a sense of codependency. These Asanas also create self-belief, self-confidence, personality independence, aspire courage and help to face the fears, and strengthen the circulatory system, heart, and brain. Asanas like headstand (Shirshasana), handstand (Adho Mukha Vrikshasana), Crow (Bakasana), opening the legs 180 degrees (Hanumanasana), etc. are some of the advanced asanas.

They are not suitable for kids of age 3-5 years old.

NOW,

Asanas and their benefits:

1- Utkatasana / Chair pose
   Strengthens the quadriceps muscles, works on pelvis – strengthens ankles.
2- Vrikshasana / Tree pose
   Improves balance, concentration and awareness – strengthens ankles – opens shoulders and rib cage – opens pelvis.
3- Garudasana / Eagle pose
   Improves balance and concentration – strengthens quadriceps muscles and ankles- Open the shoulders and stretches the trapezius muscle on the back.
4- Virabhadrasana 1 / Warrior pose 1
   Increases physical strength – opens the rib cage and lungs – stretches the back and shoulder muscles.
5- Virabhadrasana 2 / Warrior pose 2
   Strengthen legs – stretches back and stomach muscles.
6- Virabhadrasana 3 / Warrior pose 3
   Increases concentration and balance – strengthens the central muscles of the body.
7- Virasana
   Corrects flat feet – flexes the knee joint– relieves leg cramps – flexes ankles – helps with easy digestion.
8- Supta virasana

Eliminates body contractions and refreshes body – helps deeper breathing – releases heart muscles – relieves digestive problems – releases and calms the mind.

9- Gomukhasana / Cow's face pose

Eliminates crus muscle contractions – stretches shoulders and reduces back curve and hunch.

10- Navasana / boat pose

Strengthens stomach and back muscles – improves liver, kidneys and bowel function.

11- Bhujangasana / Cobra pose

Straighten the spine and work on neck and back muscles. Prevent the lower back pain.

12- Ustrasana / Camel pose

Eliminates neck and shoulders cramps.

13- Dhanurasana / Bow pose

increase flexibility in the spine – opens chest and lungs.

14- Urdhva dhanurasana / Reverse Bow pose

Corrects hunching back and droopy shoulders – improves respiratory system function – removes weakness and laziness – increases body strength and energy.

15- Kapotasana / Diamond pose

Stretches the spinal cord and increases spine flexibility – opens the chest and increases lungs capacity – inspires courage.

16- Bakasana / Crow pose

Increases awareness and concentration – strengthens stomach muscles and the central muscles of the body.

17- Bhekasana or Malasana / Frog pose

Corrects knee deviation – strengthens ankles and knees – corrects flat feet.

18- Janu sirsasana

Stretches and strengthens pelvic muscles – improves liver and lungs function – helps heart health.

19- Chaturanga Asana / Plank pose

Strengthens shoulders and arms muscles. strengthen the core.

20- Marjariasana / Cat pose

Strengthens wrist – spine flexibility – massages joints – corrects flat feet.

21- Adho mukha svanasana / Down-head dog

Strengthens leg muscles – relieves body and mind fatigue.

22- Urdhva mukha svanasana / Upward dog

Strengthens the spine and makes it flexible.

23- Chandrasana / Moon pose

Corrects flat feet – strengthens back and pelvis muscles.

24- Purvottanasana / Slide pose or table pose when with bending knees.

Corrects curvature of neck and shoulders -Realign pelvis – opens ribs and increases respiratory capacity.

25- Prasarita padottanasana

Removes fatigue – corrects tilted pelvis – open the hip joints.

26- Tadasana / Mountain pose

Helps standing correctly – stretches and strengthens the back – increases awareness.

27- Trikonasana / Triangle pose

Corrects legs deviation and strengthens ankles – corrects flat feet – strengthens chest muscles and opens rib cage.

28- Parivrtta konasana / Revolved triangle pose

Corrects lumbar flexion – corrects shoulder rotation – stretches and strengthens the core system.

29- Utthita parsvakonasana / 90 degrees triangle pose

Helps to make legs muscles and joints flexible – increases body strength.

30- Parivrtta parsvakonasana / Revolved 90 degrees triangle pose

Protects spine and reduces back pain – helps treat constipation.

31- Sirsasana / headstand pose

Releases the blood circulation toward the brain – strengthens the will power – removes fatigue and energizes – strengthens the central muscles of the body – improves immunity system – increases self-confidence.

32- Adho mukha vrksasana / Handstand pose

Strengthens the muscles of hands and wrists – strengthens shoulders muscles – increases awareness and alertness.

33- Sarvangasana / Shoulder stand pose

Affects Thyroid and Parathyroid glands – increases lungs capacity – helps fit body weight – improves gastrointestinal function – affects the immune system by simulating the Thymus gland – affects growth and general health of the body – improves headaches, colds and constipation – Glowing skin-increases freshness and calms the nervous system.

34- Halasana / Plow position

Increases flexibility and health of the spine – helps easy digestion – releases the mind and calms the body.

35- Setu Bandhasana / Bridge pose

Strengthens ankles – strengthens kidneys – strengthens spine – helps easier breathing – refreshes mind and body.

36- Surya namaskara / Relieves fatigue – affects internal body systems such as: kidneys, liver, heart and lungs – increases awareness, energizing.

***Practice:**

Now that you know about the basics of asanas and their benefits in our bodies, use your imagination and creativity to come up with some new movements you can add to your own self-created "Asanas". Design 10 new asanas by yourself.

For example, we don't have any "Ant posture", but by looking at ants and the way they move you can get inspired and create a movement and why not also design a game on it?

Watch nature, all the creatures and phenomenon, get inspired and Play!

Have Fun and I'm sure you'll come up with so many great ideas.

Write to me and let me know about your adventure.

A Summary about the Effects of Yoga on Children's Physical Challenges:

Yoga can affect some of the physical and mental challenges of childhood. Sometimes practicing from an early age can eliminate some of these challenges. Here are some good examples:

Lumbar curvature ------> strengthening waist muscles.

Stutter--------> chanting (especially group chanting), trust and cooperation games (since stutter begins from a shock or fear, these games are suitable).

Flat feet ------> Cat – Vajrasana – Ushtrasana.

Knee hyperextension ------> Utkatasana (with wall and block between the feet, leaning to the wall with completely straight back), strengthening the quadriceps muscles.

Spinal deviation (Scoliosis) --------> standing bent forward from the hip joints and staying at 90 degrees with the wall, along with pushing palms on the wall and straightening the spinal cord.

Asthma: chanting (should be brief), pulse should not rise during the exercise, opening the rib cage, Fish pose, Cobra pose, children's modified breathing movements (short, modified).

Obsession (OCD) ------> any kind of obsession including physical and intellectual, is acquired (an intellectual accumulation), for example children who don't get other children's hand during a game, etc. A way should be found to make children participate in games, for example they can take your hand if they feel comfortable with you or use a piece of fabric instead of directly taking the hand. Engaging children in games (with blindfolds, interesting and entertaining group games) moving the body, freely dancing with music, shaking, and releasing the excessive energy out.

Memory improvement ------> balancing poses.

Obesity (OBCT) -------> Sarvangasana and Halasana (if the cause is Thyroid), dynamic cycles and use of red color.

Weak wrist -------> Down-ward dog – hand balances.

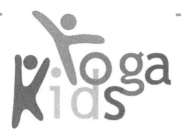

CHAPTER 11
Yoga for Special Children

You may face children who have special mental conditions or physical restrictions In your classes. In such situations, the way you deal and teach these children should be mindful of their situation. Here, some examples you may encounter are briefly presented:

Hyperactivity:

A hyperactive child is just an energetic and active child, and this is not a disorder. This child is different from those who suffer from ADHD (Attention Deficit Hyperactivity Disorder) and ADD (Attention Deficit Disorder).

You just need to be patient and help them to release their extra energies, then invite them into silence with the related games.

ADHD & ADD:

ADHD is short to (Attention Deficiency Hyperactivity Disorder) This child is an overactive child lacking attention and concentration ability. They have abrupt physical movements and may suffer from sudden jumps or tics.

In ADD, such children are not necessarily energetic and hyperactive, but they are not concentrated. They are sometimes very depressed and sometimes have high energy. They usually have many negative thoughts in their mind, don't have proper decision-making power, and may have abrupt reactions. Remember that any energetic and active child is not necessarily ADD or ADHD.

For such children, balancing poses are suitable. Yoga Nidra and the releases along with music, mental illustrations, invitation to silence and meditational games are very useful.

These children have low self-confidence since they lack concentration and are rejected by others; thus, need support and encouragement. Creative games could be useful for them.

Because of their lack of concentration and acceptance from those around them, they lack social relationships, so inviting them to cooperation and trust games, as well as pair yoga exercises, are very good for them.

Also since concentrating, copying and repeating are difficult for them, you may use the Mirror game. This game helps them to organize their minds.

Autism

Autistic children are born with this disorder. They usually become very professional in one skill. Their brain is very active on one part and inactive on other parts. For example, they can be an exceptional musician or singer but are challenged to learn other things. These children suffer from hypotension or muscles loosening. This is a very important point for a yoga instructor to know in order to make them practice within their muscle's ability. Be noted that these children usually have delay in getting the content and learning, so explanations should be very clear, and teaching should be visual. For example, if you are teaching an animal posture, showing the picture of the related animal will help. Sometimes a sense grows inside them and sometimes they might do something that might hurt them, such as self-mutilation, skin scratch, etc.

They are usually very sensitive to light, sound, etc. They are rarely understood or even ridiculed in society. Therefore, they usually lack self-confidence.

You must be very calm when dealing with them. Simple and basic asanas with full explanation and breathing games are very effective and useful for them.

Mental Retardation (Cerebral Palsy):

In this disorder, the right and left hemispheres of the brain are not balanced, and the body is deformed. Nervous system has some problems, and muscles have too much contraction. Considering that in this disorder, muscles are so stiff, gentle stretch and movement would be very useful and important for them. This disease affects medulla spinalis and spinal cord, so exercises which focus on straightening the spinal cord could be useful. Using yoga pillows or a rolled mat on the ground to massage their back is good for them. Simple twist movements and spinal massage are also useful. Since they have very little learning ability and cannot perform yoga asanas correctly, they need some simple and basic movements. Music and chanting mantra are effective in attracting their attention and learning ability. All in all, due to limitations of the movements, using devices (wall, chair, blocks, etc.) seems necessary and useful.

Down Syndrome

Children suffering from this syndrome are distinguished by their appearance. These children have both mental and physical limitations. Loose muscles (hypotonia) and very tight ligaments make stretching difficult for them. Stretching exercises should be done gently, without pressure and insistence. Moving on knees is difficult for them because their patella is weak. In this syndrome, standing is not so easy, so balancing movements are not suitable for such children, unless they get support and help. They have weak ankles and flat feet, so walking on the blade of the feet is good for them. Simple standing movements are also suitable for strengthening their feet.

They usually have problems with digestion and their gastrointestinal system; they are often constipated, so twist movements could be effective and pleasant for them. Using music, free style dancing, singing, and chanting are among other suitable alternatives for this group of children.

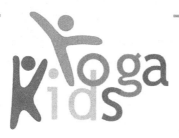

CHAPTER 12
Creative Games

In such games, we mostly use children's creativity and imagination, as well as their cooperation with each other in a group.

You can choose a theme and story, then build your session upon the subject.

You start your session with a story. Always find stories which have some moral learning in it. You 'll find some samples in this section.

You can give them a short visualization on imagining your theme and taking them into picturing the journey in their minds.

Then follow up with your story, adding your asanas and games in it.

Then Always finish the session with taking them into a reminder of what they learned with your guided voice in Savasana.

By the way, bear in mind that any group game which is introduced in other chapters can be added in your designed sessions depending on your theme and your creative process of designing your session.

Here we'll go through some creative subjects, themes and stories for you to have an idea about how you can get inspired and create a fun session with lots of creative games, moral lessons, effective asanas, relaxation,...

1. Letters and numbers

Stand in a circle and ask the children to move in a circular way. First begin with yourself standing in the middle of the circle. Close your eyes and bring one arm forward pointing at children in the circle and start to turn around repeating sentences like "Go...go...go! Faster, faster! Slower, slower!" This will give energy to the children to walk, run or whatever idea you come up with at that time. After a while, say, "Stop!" The children should all stop. Then ask the child who you are pointing at randomly to form the shape of a number or letter of the alphabet with their body. They can use one of the asanas known to them or anything they can think of. Then ask everyone to try. The chosen child goes into the middle of the circle and the game continues until everyone has had the opportunity to be in the middle once.

Variations on the game:

* Write a name on a board and ask the children to make the shapes of the letters with their bodies.

* Ask a child to spell a name with their body for the others to guess.

* Divide the children into two separate groups. Each group chooses a sentence. The group will perform the sentence, each child being a letter, and the other group has to read the sentence. Then switch the groups.

* All children stand in one line. Hearing a bell, they should walk among each other and change their place fast. With the next bell sound, everyone stands wherever they are and makes a Latin letter. Together we guess the letters one by one and take a note of them. Now we divide the children to two groups and ask them to make a few meaningful words with the created letters. This has a very huge impact on the child's creativity, accuracy, and attention.

2. Imagine a jungle

First try to create a sense of being in a jungle by telling them a story about a jungle. Ask them to sit in silence for a couple of minutes and imagine themselves being an animal. Ask them to choose an animal that they'd like to be and sound a bell to invite them out of silence. They can then become their imaginary animal. After a couple of minutes, ring the bell again and they should freeze! They can also look around to see the other animals. Then ask them to guess what the other animals are. If a child's animal identity is correctly guessed that child must sit out of the game, while the remaining animals play a couple more rounds, following the same pattern. Once they have played for a while, imagining to be and act like all the beings in a jungle, tell them that we are now going to learn the yoga way of being all these beings which exist in a jungle, and start to teach them some of the asanas which exist in a jungle. You can continue this game in different sessions, and each time teach them a new asana from the jungle. When you ask them to lie down and go into Savasana, you can play music with the sound of the jungle and close the session with the feeling that they have been on a journey into a magical jungle! Then ask them to share their experience with the group.

The lion's birthday party, with a cake and candles on it

Choose a child as the lion of the jungle. If it's a child's birthday, it's nice to make them the lion of the jungle. The remaining children are the candles on the cake. Ask the children to lie down on their mats in a circle and then guide them to go to shoulder stand posture (Sarvangasana). You will instruct them how to do this before starting the game. In this position, they'll look like the candles on the cake. Keep in mind that younger children do this pose naturally but normally, not with a straight spine. As the lion blows out the candles one by one, the children move into Halasana position and roll back from the exercise slowly.

Use music which includes the sounds of a jungle.

Other Variations of the exercise:

- Each child in turn becomes an animal and the others guess what animal it is.

- You may teach the asana related to different jungle animals after everyone imitates an animal out of their imagination.

Here are some examples of different subjects. You may make these shapes in children's bodies, using yoga asanas along with your own creativity. You may even ask them, for example, what they think a squirrel looks like. Ultimately, you may use an asana most similar to your subject, by slightly changing it. Also, for starting the class and the ending Savasana you may design a class by using the same theme.

Jungle animals and Freeze game:

Play a piece of music with a jungle background and sounds. Ask children to walk and move around the classroom and make animals, plants and anything that might be found in the jungle, with their bodies. Then stop the music and everyone has to freeze in the shape they are. Now children should guess each other's posed animal. Anyone who guesses correctly gets free from the pose. This goes on until all children are free. This game can be played several times. Obviously, this game cultivates children's creativity and imagination.

How to perform some creative movements based on different animals and creatures existing in the imaginary jungle:

Squirrel: Sitting on toes, holding hands in front of the chest and wrinkling the nose!

Giraffe: Tadasana (standing), pulling hands above the head like the long neck of a giraffe and putting the palms on each other.

Kangaroo: Utkatasana on the soles of the feet and jumping.

Wolf: walking in Adomhukhashvanasana and roaring.

Bear: Adomhukhashvanasana with open legs and hands

Monkey: Hanumanasana.

Unicorn: Ustrasana and pulling hands backwards and above the head in Garudasana position.

Upside down trees: Adomhukhashvasana.

Robin Hood: Warrior 1 and 2

Lion: Simhasana.

3- Using the theme of Lake:

You can come out with a story about Lake and take them into a journey by a lake and play with what you can find beside a lake!

You can always start your class, by gathering the kids, using the train game or cars to take the road to go to the lake side...

You can play the Frog race & use the frog song.

Then take them into different postures and even a vinyasa flow using different creatures you'll find by a lake such as bellow:

Frog: Malasana.

Flamingo: Natarajasana.

Alligator: Chaturanga Asana.

Crocodile: Chaturanga Dandasana.

Lilies: Padmasana.

Swan: Dhanurasana.

Boat: Navasana.

Mosquito: Virasana and elbows upwards along with buzzing sound.

Lizard: Nakarasana.

Komodo dragon: walking in Makarasana position.

You can add some fun games and the moral story of the crocodile brother, you'll be introduced to later in this chapter.

4- Imagining the ocean:

Like the jungle game, start by painting the picture of an ocean in their mind by visually guiding them but also show them some pictures or some information you gather about the ocean and play the same game with all the beings in the ocean. To help them imagine being in the ocean, it's a good idea to use the bubble meditation, which allows them to feel safe and protected. You can also use dolphins as their friends through the journey (in order for them to not get scared) especially at the end when you finish the class with a short yoga nidra, imagining an ocean.

>What we can find in an Ocean theme:

Crab: walking in Poroutanasana.

Starfish: sleeping on the back along with opening and closings the limbs (suitable for Savasana).

Shark: various Shalabhasanas, hooking hands behind.

Wale: various Shalabhasanas, opening the limbs.

Dolphin: Adomhukhashvanasana on forearm.

Turtle: Kurmasana.

Seashell: bending forward in Bakasana pose.

Fish: Matsyasana.

Sea horse: Ushtrasana, hands in Garudasana pose.

Boat: Navasana.

Wave: making waves with wavy movements of hands/Adomhukhashvanasana, making waves in the spine/standing and making waves in the whole body.

Jellyfish: Navasana with open limbs and making wavy movements, floating in the waves.

Mermaid: this pose could be made like a cycle in a row, such that the mermaid sits on the beach in Gomukhasana pose. In that same pose, she makes Adomhukhashvanasana and moves her body, meaning that she is swimming. Also, in the same cross feet position, showing her tail, she makes urdhva Mukha Svanasana, meaning that she gets out her head from the water. Then again, she sits on the beach in Gomukhasana pose.

Group octopus: all children sit in a row, open their legs and hands and start moving them continuously balancing in their bottoms. If you take a picture from the front of the front row It looks like an octopus!

5- Imagining seasons:

You can create a sense of a season every session and play games relating to the chosen season. For example, if you choose the autumn, bring some colourful leaves to class and do breathing exercises with the leaves. Or for spring time, you could use the massage exercise to simulate rain on their backs using the fingers (tapping).

At the end of the class, you can play Vivaldi's "Four seasons" during savasana.

6- The story of "Seven Cities of Love" by Attar and imagining different birds:

First tell them the mythical story of "Seven Cities of Love", by the Persian poet Attar Neishaboori. Use your creativity and encourage them to move their bodies into different kinds of birds they hear in the story...

The story is as follows:

One day lots of beautiful birds gathered together and decided to search for the King of the birds who were better, more beautiful and more complete than any other bird. A bird named Simurgh (a combination of Si=30 and Murgh=bird)!

They started the journey. They went far away. They flew as far as they could. Some of them got tired and stopped in the middle of the way. But some others searched seven cities of love all over. This searching grew more difficult at each stage, and each time some of the birds refused to continue flying. Only 30 birds remained in the seventh city. They looked everywhere for Simurgh but tired, confused and thirsty, they decided to go to the lake and drink some water. When the image of the 30 birds fell in the water, all of a sudden one of them understood that Simurgh (30 birds) is them; the best and most complete of them.

The best of us is inside us. We also find Simurgh when we unite and stay together in hardship and go through them; be together and grow together.

You may also use the same themes of birds and start your session by a moral lesson such as cooperation, friendship, togetherness...and at the end of the session remind them of what the story inspires us and maybe you can give them a little note or a practice related to the subject so that they can think about till their next session.

Different Birds:

The bird of paradise asana: Svarga Dvijasana

Pigeon: Akapadarajkaputasana.

Owl: We sit on toes, make two rings with our fingers, put them on our eyes like the owl's big eyes, and turn our head to right and left.

Crow: Bakasana.

Crain: In standing position, we bend forward with straight back and straight knees. Take the ankle of one foot with both hands, separate the other foot from the ground, straightly pull it back and up, and stay in a balancing position.

Flamingo: Natarajasana.

Swan: Dhanurasana.

Peacock: Mayorasana.

Eagle: Garudasana.

Peacock: Pinchamayorasana.

7- The Ugly Duckling story and performing types of swan movement:

This story is also among the beautiful and influential stories you can dedicate a session to. You can tell and play this story by talking about the fact that everyone is beautiful in their own way, we are all just different and no one is superior to others: "There was an ugly duckling absolutely different from others. It was born in a family that bore no resemblance to other members in appearance. It thought it was ugly and ungainly. It didn't know it was a different bird. It was not a duckling at all, but it was a cygnet who had been settled among the duck eggs when it was just an egg. When it grew up, it became a beautiful magnificent swan."

(Swan can be shown as Dhanurasana posture. You can add its variations such as going to the left, the right. one leg, on hand up, then change the hand & Leg,...)

Then you can explain that being different is not being ugly. All of us are beautiful in our own way and have differences with others.

This story is especially influential on children with special physical problems.

Using your creativity and imagination, you may take children to different trips with similar different stories. Using their imagination and creativity, you can invite them into different asanas during the game.

Let's continue with some more fun themes:

8-Insects theme:

Glowworm: Shalabhasana.

Dragonfly: Shalabhasana with open hands and completely paired feet.

Spider: Doing Dhanurasana with the wall.

Silkworm: Transformation of cocoon to worm, from Virasana to Bhujangasana.

Butterfly: Badakunasana.

Cocoon: Virasana.

Worm: Bhujangasana with hands clinging to the sides.

Mosquito: Virasana, taking elbows up from the sides and making a buzz sound.

Ladybug: Virasana, bending the arms from elbow, taking wrists at the sides and flapping with hands.

Grasshopper: Shalabhasana.

Scorpion: Vrishchikasana.

Millipede: We sit in a row like a train, bend our knees, put our feet on the groin of the front person, put our hands next to our body on the ground, and separate our legs and pelvis from the ground with the press of the hands, and collectively move back and forth on our hands.

9-Desert:

Pyramids: Triangle posture (Trikonasana)

Sphinx: Sphinx pose.

Scorpion: Vrishchikasana.

Camel: Ushtrasana.

Snake: Bhujangasana

Mummy: The child horizontally lies down on the mat. Gently roll her with the mat the way the mat wraps around her and she takes the shape of a mummy. This game is suitable for children over 6 years of age.

The beautiful Starry sky night of the desert: Lying in savasana

10-Food stuff:

Baguette Sandwich: Paschimottanasana.

Jelly: Moving and shaking the body in lying position (suitable for Savasana).

Popcorn: Jumping from sitting to standing position like corn kernels which open abruptly and loudly.

Pineapple: Sitting on the soles of the feet and putting hands above the head like the pineapple crown.

Falafel: Sitting in Virasana pose and getting round like falafels.

Pizza: Sitting in Opavishtakunasan pose and imagining the pizza dough between our legs, with stretched back and straight knees; in all positions we move our trunk to right and left, so that we perform the asana correctly and completely during the game. We use imaginary food stuff and at the same position, we bake an imaginary pizza.

Cake: It is like making a pizza.

Sushi: Wrapping the mat around the child (like the Mummy pose).

Donut: Badakunasana with an open angle knees.

Spaghetti or noodles: This exercise is useful for relaxation and before Savasana. While the child is lying down, take the child's legs and pull them up. Ask her to relax her body and put her weight to your hands. Now move the legs the way all her body moves and her back stretches. Then, gently put her feet on the ground and leave them there.

11-Story telling:

We are fascinated by stories. It is an easy way to focus children and keep the yoga class interesting. Invite them into stories using a book that has possible yoga poses, or using your own imagination and creativity. The children too can help as they create stories in their mind. This can be encouraged by starting the class with a story and letting them add to it. They can also be encouraged to learn different asanas while they are playing the games.

Be playful and at the same time be decisive. Discipline becomes an issue when the teacher is unclear about their limits or cannot communicate them in a positive way. Kids feel more relaxed and more trusting when they know that the teacher is in charge and can efficiently deal with any issues that may arise. So create your boundaries and stick to them. This means creating your own set of rules, as well as the rules created together with the children, and not breaking them. If you break your own rules, the children will learn that there are no rules and they can do whatever they want.

12-Drawing a Mandala:

Mandala is a sacred geometric shape helping to improve your concentration and increases your mind power. When we draw or paint a Mandala or even just stare at it, without thinking of anything or trying to empty the mind, we get into a meditation pose. Children love drawing and painting. We may use this enthusiasm, encourage them to do yoga exercises and paint Mandala.

The word Mandala is taken from the ancient Sanskrit language and means a symbolic ring. Mandala is the symbol of the essence of our existence, since we can see them in all stages of our lives. We live on the earth planet, which along with other planets, stars, galaxies and the whole universe have a permanent swirl around themselves and around the Sun. We move the same as the stars, in the family, friends and society circle. All living creatures on the earth are made from cells. Each cell has a nucleus. This central nucleus is the beginning of a Mandala; the central nucleus of a circle. If we take each atom as a Mandala, we would find out that mandalas exist everywhere around us in the world; in flowers, seas, fruits, snowflakes, etc. Everywhere! Open your eyes and look at your surroundings. Where you can find mandalas? Anything that has a center with extensions inward and outward, is an evolution which is called mandala.

You may also create a **"human mandala"** with performing group yoga asanas. Different beautiful shapes can be made with group yoga asanas done in a circle.

You can put one kid or a smaller group of kids in the middle of the circle and the other around a bigger circle, then ask them to perform a collaborative dance of asanas together, shaping a group mandala.

Human mandalas may be settled and imobile, or better moving; In a way that you may play with the shapes of asanas by changing and transforming them.

As an example:

Have a small group sitting in the middle of the centre in Dandasana.

Then the bigger circle around them will sit in Upavistha Konasana.

Play soft music and then ask the bigger group to start by rising their hands and going up & down while the inner circle stays in dandasan.

Then ask the outer circle to stay with their hands on their inner thighs, and ask the inner circle to raise their arms and go back and forth into paschimottanasana.

It will also look like a Kaleidoscope!

You can also call it "Kaleidoscope yoga"!

Play with creating plenty of human mandalas! It is so much fun, looks so beautiful and you can even arrange a performance for their parents and friends.

Introducing mandala to children:

1- One session before you are going to teach mandala, ask the children to take colored pencils, pastels, etc. to the class for the next session (unless you have already arranged enough of them in the classroom).

2- Play soft and pleasant music and sit round in a circle.

3- Take a flower or a fruit with you to the class (orange, apple, kiwi and....). Ask the children where inside or outside of the classroom they can see a mandala.
Attract their attention to the circle they are sitting in, and tell them that they themselves have created a mandala. Cut the fruits from the middle and show them the mandala inside it. Ask them where they can see a mandala either inside or outside the room: in eyes, face, top of the head, navel and …..

4- Now it is the time to paint mandalas (You can bring some images of mandalas suitable for their age group, as a sample to show them before they start drawing.)

5- Guide the children to observe the following rules:

a) Please keep quiet and stay concentrated.

b) Don't look at your friends' mandalas (you may make them sit back to back, or sit in a circle one facing to the center and the next facing outwards and so and forth).

c) Paint your mandala in the quietest state you can. Give them some estimated time and ask them to try to finish before the time is up. You can always tell them that: If your painting is not finished in the class, you may take it home with you, and finish it there then bring it with you next time for us to see.

6- You can then tell them:

Now that you have created your own mandala, you may put them wherever inside the classroom or at home, and use it as a device for meditation, concentration or relaxation; you get positioned in front of it, take a deep breath and stare at the center of the mandala. Now let your thoughts get out of your head one by one. Slowly by slowly look deeper into the center of the mandala and unite with the love and harmony that is surrounding you.

13-Nature Kid:

The theme is to look at natural phenomenons in nature and play with creating the shape of it in their bodies.

Storm: running around the classroom while blowing at each other and making the sound of a storm. This movement could be used as warm up or when the class needs energy release.

Volcano: start in sitting position with the knees bent inside the stomach and the head between the hands. Now we all erupt, jump up with a sound, stand, open hands and legs.

Rain: getting in Utkatasana pose, we all tap on our stomachs, chests, thighs and make the sound of raining.

Earthquake: shaking the whole body in standing position.

Fire: round in a circle in Dandasana pose, we get hands above the head and move them up and down, left and right like flames.

Wave: making waves with wavy movements of the hands / Adomukhashvanasana and making waves in the spine / standing and making waves in the whole body.

Tornado: spinning in standing position along with the sound of tornado.

Rainbow: Vasisthasana, raising hand, moving it in crescent form and moving pelvis up and down.

Thunderbolt: doing Virabhadrasana 3, moving to right and left and making the sound of a thunder.

Lunar eclipse: Chandrasana and Arkham Chandrasana.

Eclipse of the sun: sitting together in a circle in Dandasana pose and making Paschimottanasana which means we have covered the sun!

14- Going to a park:

You can design a session in which you take children to a theme park. For example, a tour in the city a part of which is dedicated to going to a theme park. For making a small theme park you may use the following asanas:

Slide: Purvottanasana or Adomukhashvanasana.

Swinging: two children take the hands and feet of one child and swing her.

Theme park train: Utkatasana and standing in one queue.

Merry-go-round: Divide children to two groups with one group standing in a circle and the other group sitting one by one on the ground between them in the same circle, with their feet on a soft fabric or towel right in the middle of the circle. They get each other's hands, and those who are standing, start rotating the circle. The group which is sitting should strongly hold their feet on the fabric. Of course the type of floor mat is very important in this game. The less the friction there is, the easier the children slide. You may add variety to this game, for example, the sitting group gets into Purvottanasana or Navasana pose with the fabric under their pelvis, stick their legs together in the middle space of the circle, and play the game above the ground level.

Children enjoy playing this game so much that you may have to come with ticks so that they don't want to repeat it again and again!

Then, they change places and continue. This game is full of excitement, laughter and joy. Using your creativity, you may design other games for your theme park and enjoy creating lots of exciting moments to play along with kids.

15- A Tour in the city game:

This game can also cover one whole session of your class. Start and end of the class could be dedicated to the city, living in it and promoting the environmental culture. Then, like "A Trip to India" game, first they get into a bus, then an urban train, after that an elevated railroad and finally they pass through a tunnel! (A group makes a tunnel in a queue in Down-head Dog pose and the others pass under it either on their fours or crawling). Ultimately, after playing different games in the city, they may get into a Shavasana pose which is named The **Train of Laughter**, the way that one child lies down, the next one puts her head on the previous one's stomach and like this, they all get into Savasana, by clinging to each other. First, they would laugh a lot from the movement of each other's heads and hear the growling of each other's stomachs, but finally they get relaxed with each other's breaths, close their eyes and follow your guided voice into relaxation.

16-North Pole:

For this theme, I'm going to take you first into an inspiring story, which you may tell it in the class and then spend some time in the snow, ice and beautiful sky of the north pole by introducing different asanas.

The story is as follows:

"Otek and the old whale"

"There was a tender-hearted, Eskimo boy named "Otek" but because he was very kind, everybody called him wimpy. Days passed and Otek grew bigger until he got married. One day he was searching for food when he suddenly saw a big old whale stuck in the ice. This whale could supply his family's food for a long time. The whale realized what he was thinking about and told him: "Wait, don't kill me. I am an old whale and will shortly die. Please let my life end in peace."

The boy replied:

Why not? You are plenty of food for my children and your oil can warm our house.

The whale continued: If you help me and refuse to kill me, I promise that I will make up for your kindness.

Otek's heart pounded and trusted the whale. He broke the ice and rescued it. The whale told him: "I will see you again…! Thank you for your kindness!

When Otek got back home and told the story, his wife started to shout, and blamed him for his mistake. But his children believed him. A few months passed and Otek became disappointed and depressed; he realized that he could no longer keep his house warm and provide for his family. Then One day he went hopelessly to the ocean where he met the whale again. The whale moved its tail strongly in the water and thousands of fish sprang up around Otek. There were as many fish as his family's one year food supply.

Otek took the fish home and they celebrated together. He was rewarded for his kind heart as promised by the whale.

Otek had a heart as big as an old whale…!

Eskimo: Tadasana.

Igloo: in standing, opening the legs 3 times, shoulders distance apart and raining the arms up as the palms join together.

Fish: Matsiasana.

Kayak: Navasana

Whale: Shalabhasana with open limbs.

Polar bear: Adomukhashvanasana with open limbs.

Walrus: lion breathing in Salabhasana pose.

Seal: Shalabhasana with hands clinging to the body.

Seagull: Akapadarajkaputtasana.

Setting fire: we settle down in a circle in a Dandasana pose, raise hands and move them up and down, left and right like fire flames. Rub the palms together and warm ourselves. Also give a group massage and warm each other.

Penguin: we stand on the knees, bend legs from back and raise them slightly. It is better to do this on a soft mat to avoid hurting the knees. Now we try to walk on the knees like the short legs of a penguin.

17-The Magical Sunflower game:

We invite the children to sit in a circle. You may start by guiding them first to sit with a straight back and a happy smile on their face while opening the chest like a happy, shiny sun!

You all together look like a magical, big, colorful sunflower!

You may begin to ask them to choose a color and each can also have a magic power through which they can share their sparks into the circle during the game!

Then you can take them into different postures as explained below to open the circle of the magical sunflower!

You need to keep reminding them of these points throughout the game:

- Keep your bag straight
- Open your chest and have a big shiny smile from your heart
- Keep breathing deeply through your nose while going into a posture, then deeply breath out when releasing
- Keep a happy smile on your beautiful face!

- They can sit in Badhokansana pose (Butterfly), and place the soles of their feet together. Then open the feet apart from each other like an open book and start reading the book.

You can play by asking them what kind of book they are reading?

- Take one ankle with the opposite hand and pull it upward toward the shoulders, and start playing a guitar, like the toes are the guitar strings. Ask them to take their knees as high as they can while having their back straight.

- They can hug their legs in their chest as if they are hugging a baby and by rocking, puting it to sleep. They can even sing lullabies for their baby!

- Or bring the sole of one foot close to their ear and act like they are talking on the phone.

- Take a ball between the feet, pass it to the next one, without using hands, and rotate the ball cautiously with their feet through the circle.

- Stretch their legs while sitting in the circle, and get into Dandasana pose the way all the soles stick together in the center of the circle, just as they are the seeds of the magical sunflower. Now imagine that they are a big magical colorful sunflower. You may make a variety of sitting positions in sunflower pose with them and enjoy. For example, Paschimutanasana and catching the toes of friends in the center of the circle, opening and closing the flower, moving to right and left, performing Navasana and sticking the soles of the feet together in the center of the circle, Shavasana in the same circle position and touching the feet, etc.

- Don't forget that your main goal is to introduce yoga asanas, so during the game emphasize on the Open Sun Smile, straight back and other important points of each asana.

18-The Crocodile games:

Games with the subject of crocodile are Fun, energetic games you may play & use it in your lake and jungle theme or just teach the related postures, you can talk about the differences between a crocodile and alligator as an example, give some informations about the species then play the games along with them.

Before explaining the games, here is an inspiring story with a great message:

The King of the Crocodiles had 7 sons. One day he summoned his sons and said: "Whoever of you that can make me happy by bringing me something I need, I will give my crown to him and he will be my successor.

The first son gave him 7 pearls inside a seashell, but unfortunately the seashell stuck to his hand and caused him pain and discomfort.

The second son gave him 7 rubies. The King Crocodile thought they were cherries; ate them and broke all his teeth.

The third son gave him 7 lemon seeds but the king said: "Lemon seeds are of no use to me because I have no teeth."

The fourth sun gave him 7 cuckoo clocks on which there was the figure of a beautiful dancer, but the sound of the clock annoyed the king.

The fifth son gave him 7 bottles of fragrant perfumes, but different fragrances mixed and caused him a headache.

The sixth son gave him 6 diamond rings but since crocodiles walk on their hands and feet, the rings got stuck and caused the king to fall.

The seventh son came to his father and said: "Father it seems that you need help so he hugged him and helped him get up from the ground. The King Crocodile told the seventh son: "Son, You might not have given me anything but You will be my successor because you gave me your hand in support when I needed you…!

The moral of the story is that, The best gift you can give to anyone is your help and support.

1- Ask the children to get settled in a circle and lie on their stomachs. They have the role of the river crocodiles; as they are lying, they open and close their legs from behind, like a crocodile's mouth. One child should pass through this river and be watchful not to get stuck in the crocodiles' mouths. She should step forward before the crocodiles' mouths close and cross the path forward without getting stuck in their mouths (meaning the feet should not touch the moving legs). If she gets stuck, she should change her place with the one who caught her. You may ask children to open and close their legs slowly at first and speed up in next turns so that the game becomes more challenging to them.

2- Ask some of the children to lie on the ground next to each other so that their hips are in line. Then they will join their palms together and stretch their arms above their heads and join their feet together. They all form lying crocodiles, helping one crocodile to cross the lake!

   Then one child who is the crossing crocodile, will stand in front of the line where all the bottoms are joined together in one line. She will gently dive in! You can also ask for 3 more friends, helping by lifting hey and gently placing her on the crocodile queue.

   Ask the lying children to roll over at the same time so that the child on top of them moves forward and crosses a pond full of the crocodiles.

3- Put some chocolates, candies (Try to choose the more healthy ones!;)), colored balls or anything you want in the middle of the circle. All children get positioned in Sphinx mode in a circle. With the sound of a bell, the children move toward the candies in the same position, like crocodiles walking. Everyone takes one candy or chosen item each time and brings it back, and again moves toward the center for fetching the next candy. Finally, the one who collects more candies is a sharper and smarter crocodile but in the condition of respecting all the game rules.

19-Play dough:

Items needed: A few packets of playdough – paper or cardboard

Ask the children to get into groups of two. One makes the asana with her body and the other one tries to make a statue from her with the play dough. Use the paper or cardboard as the plate on which the statue is made. This game could be used for inviting silence, learning about asanas and doing self adjustment in the posture by posing, as well as fostering creativity.

Other variation of the game:

You may ask the children to sit in a circle. One of them becomes a model and poses as an asana in the middle of the circle, and the others make her statue with the playdoughs. At the end, you may hold a small exhibition of their art pieces and invite the parents to visit it.

20-Animal mix:

Items needed: cards of animals pictures.

Ask the children to close their eyes and sit quietly in a circle. Tell them that they are going to turn into magical machines; something like a washing machine! which mix 2 animals and creates a new invented animal!

Put 2 cards with the picture of animals on each person's lap while they have their eyes closed and tell them: "Now I have put 2 cards inside the machine. Open your eyes and look at your cards without letting anyone see the pictures on them; two different animals!" Then after they saw their cards, ask them to close their eyes again and hug themselves, which means they have closed the door of the machine. Now ask them to move their bodies to right and left. This means they mix the animals inside the machine. Now that they pictured the image of the new creature mixed while they were swinging, invite them to go to a created posture and show the result in their bodies, still keeping their eyes closed! This is a new creature which has the properties of both animals.

When all of them showed their new creature, ask them to open their eyes and guess each other's mixed animals. Guess which two animals were used to create this new mixture! Anyone who's animals have been guessed correctly will be released from the pose.

21-Music Orchestra

You may design one session based on music and musical instruments; The theme will be an orchestra!

Children can imitate different instruments with their bodies, through different asanas and all together they will make a big orchestra!

Each child may play the role of an instrument; you guide them and compose a music orchestra as the conductor. The conductor is responsible for the health of instruments so that they don't break or spoil. The rib cage is open and asanas are performed completely and correctly. Here, some examples on the instruments you can use are presented. Be creative, use your imagination and take them into a magnificent orchestra!

- Drum: Utkatasana and tapping with hand on legs and body.

- Guitar: sitting in Dandasana pose, embracing one leg and playing guitar.

- Piano: tapping on the ground with toes in Tadasana pose.

- Saxophone: making hand Garudasana, making sound with the mouth.

- Violin: taking one foot in Dandasana, opening the pelvis and moving the bow by hand.

- Flute: moving with hand and making sound (respiratory exercise)

- Orff: playing the instrument with toes, while the legs are gathered inside the belly and the feets are on the ground.

- Trumpet: Navasana with bent and straight legs, making bass sound with the mouth.

- Accordion: opening the hands to sides with inhalation and closing hands with exhalation (breathing exercise).

- Tar: same as guitar.

Nobieh Kiani fard

- Dulcimer: Badakunasana and playing the instrument with hands.

- Tonbak: tapping on the stomach.

- vocal: singing.

Variety of the game: divide children to two groups. Each group is a music band and has a leader; together they select some musical instruments. Then give them a chance to collaborate together and prepare a piece of music to play. Now each group performs for the other group.

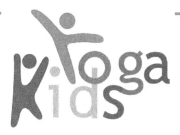

CHAPTER 13
Cooperation and Trust Games

In this section, we point to games which teach children how to cooperate and trust each other while playing. When others trust you and reveal their weaknesses to you, there emerges a pleasant feeling which makes you feel responsible for them. When you trust others, you find this courage to reveal your true emotions and weaknesses, you feel no need to defend yourself against them, but you can consider them as friends who support you and actually you feel free to be yourself around them without any guilt or shame.

This way you will be able to say bravely "NO", when you find yourself in unpleasant situations.

Being aware of personal limitations and respecting others' boundaries and limitations are among the goals of such games mentioned in this section. If there is no mutual trust between the children in the class yet, it is better not to offer such games, and you should be very sensitive in choosing the right game at the right time.

It is very important to establish the trust step by step. In choosing such types of games, The first priority is to build a sense of trust among them.

After playing these games, you should talk to the children about their experience, and getting inspired from their ideas and suggestions, you may coordinate and harmonize the games with the level of understanding of kids in their age group.

In the school:

Nowadays children are individually involved in many activities, and they spend lots of time by themselves. They sit in front of a computer alone, ipads, iphones or watch television alone,

Or maybe with their small circles, but each of them travels in their own world. In the school, the focus is mostly on their grades and they are constantly judged by their achievements or lack of it.

In this environment, children learn to continuously compare themselves and compete with others. Some even try to make themselves look better by humiliating others. Sometimes children behave with others very viciously without knowing. Unfortunately, despising others is seen among children very often. Using these exercises, children learn to trust each other, recognize their boundaries and respect them, take responsibility and understand each other. By learning these games in yoga class, they can practice them in the school, during break time, with other children as well as their friends.

1. Guide & Walk

Items needed: Blindfolds.

In this game, divide children into groups of pairs. In each group, one child wears a blindfold and the other plays the role of a guide. The role of each child is specified; the first one should trust the second and the second one should take the responsibility of the first. The guide has the role of a supporter and must take care of the blindfolded one not to hit anything.

Select the groups of pairs, one of them either wears a blindfold or closes her eyes. The other one holds the blindfolded child's hands and shoulders, and they walk together around the classroom. It is better if the guide holds the blindfolded child's shoulders so that she walks by herself and just feels that someone is guiding her from behind. The guide can announce, in advance, which direction they are moving.

For example: "We turn a little right because there is a chair and a table in front of us."

Then ask the two children in the group to shift their roles. Shifting roles causes both of them to experience the sense of support. After doing the exercise, ask them to talk about their feelings and experience.

Different variations of the game:

The guide doesn't touch the other kid, instead verbally guides her during the walk.

The guide stays behind the other kid by touching her shoulders and taking her into different spaces in the room.

- The guide takes the hand of the blindfolded child and takes her to different sides of the room. Then ask them about the differences between this mode and the previous one.

You may play this game with groups of three as well, such that one wears a blindfold and the two others take her shoulders together, and guide her to move around the classroom.

It is better for children between 3 to 5 years of age not to close their eyes, and it is enough to guide each other from behind.

- You can add some objects such as a table, chairs or foam yoga blocks...in the classroom, you may make the game more interesting so that the blindfolded child can pass under the table or turn around the chair, jump from the yoga block, with the help of the guide.

2. Moving Backward

In this game, one child moves backward, while the other one guides her. Since we cannot see behind us, some children find it difficult and are sometimes afraid. The child should trust that the other one guides her to the correct and safe direction. The guide should be confident & responsible enough to guide her partner in a secure way.

This game develops a sense of trust, cooperation, and awareness of the environment in children.

Divide children into groups of pairs. One child stands with her back to the wall and the other child stands facing the opposite wall of the class with her back to the first child. The child who stands facing the wall should move backwards to the wall behind her and the other child must guide her. For example: "I got you. Let's go. You are doing well. Now go a little to the left not to hit Sarah...." Then the roles shift.

Another mode of the game:

- The child who is moving backwards is blindfolded or closed-eyed. (Only for kids over 8 years old)

3. Dancing together

Items needed: Blindfolds and soft music.

In this game, same as the previous one, children are divided into groups of pairs. One of them wears a blindfold and the other, guides the dance by holding her hands (without exchanging any word).

The blindfolded child should pay attention to the guide's movements and try to adjust to the rhythm of her movement. In this game you should definitely use soft music.

Music creates rhythm and encourages the child to move. The blindfolded one learns to listen to the music more carefully, and adjust herself to the movements of the other child, and the other child should try to make her understand how to dance by giving hints; move ahead, back, slowly, fast and…Ask the children to change their roles and dance together again.

Other variations of the game:

- The guide can use words to tell the other child how to move.

- When children get to know this game, you can use more rhythmic music.

4. The Mirror

-Music is helping in this game.

In this game, the two playmates should imitate each other's movement while the palms of their hands are touching. The hands that come in contact with each other create a sense of cooperation in this game. The two playmates should have sufficient concentration and attention in their movements.

Ask the children to stay in front of their partner. bring their hands in front of their chest while palms are touching.

One plays the role of a mirror and the other plays the role of the person in front of the mirror. The one playing the person looking at the mirror, moves her hands and the other one follows her movement. The palms of their hands keep the contact.

Other variations of the game:

- The one who has the role of the mirror closes her eyes.

- Both children play with closed eyes.

- Children play this game while they are sitting, and the soles of their feet are in contact with each other.

5. The Group hug

All children stand next to each other and hold hands. From one end of the line, one child stands as the center and doesn't move. The first child on the other end of the line begins to move and the others follow her while still holding each other's hands. They move or run around the fixed child and continue this until all of them make a big circular hug. Two children can stand in turn in the middle or at the end of the line. This game can be used to create a warmer and more intimate atmosphere in the classroom.

6. The Group Knot

The number of children should definitely be more than 5 in this game. Ask them to stand in a circle. Each child stretches her arms in front of her, then crosses one arm over the other and each hand will take a hand of a different child in front of the circle.

Now we have a knotted circle!

Then, without letting go of their hands for even a second, they will try to open the knots by moving their bodies and at the end they will turn into a circle again!

This game needs lots of collaboration, wise moves by listening to each other and also the body is moving in many different ways and works on flexibility. It's fun and also inspires a sense of trust, friendship and problem solving in a team and group work.

7. Guiding the group

Items needed: yoga blocks – blindfold – yoga mat.

In this game, you set some objects in the classroom which can be the yoga blocks and rolled mats.

It goes this way:

You arrange a few lines with the yoga blocks or rolled yoga mats. You can also do a mixture of both.

you'll have some lines as barriers.

depending on the number of kids this game can play in one or few different groups.

All kids from one group will stand in a line parallel to the barriers.

One kid will be the group leader, who'll guide her team member into crossing the barriers.

The guide will be in the middle and all of them will hold each other's arm so that all of them have their arms clasp together and they will move altogether at the same time without detaching their arms from one another.

Now, All kids will be blindfolded except the Guide situated in the middle.

When they hear the starting bell, They will move forward by crossing over the borders.

The guide is the one to arrange the group movements, so that they can step over the borders, without touching any block or yoga mats.

For example she says: "Everyone stand, hold up your right leg and take one step forward. Now put your right foot on the ground, and slowly put your left foot beside it."

In this game, a sense of responsibility and trust grows in children.

Make sure all of them become the guide once. If there are too many kids, better to play this game in different sessions so that everyone experiences the feeling of being the guide and responsible for a group.

Other variations you can add:

- Instead of taking steps, jumping can be used, or instead of moving forward, moving backward.

8. Gathering the Balls

Items needed: some small balls (you can use tennis balls) – blindfold – bags or baskets.

Divide children into two groups to stand in a row in two different queues, and put their hands on each other's shoulders or waists. All but the last one in the queue, who is the group guide, should be blindfolded. Throw the balls on the ground, and consider a bag or a basket for each group, which you have already put at a corner of the class for each group separately. In this game, no word should be exchanged and each group should set some conventional points for conveying a message. For example, a tap on the right shoulder means turn to the right, or pushing shoulders means sit and…The last one whose eyes are open conveys the message to the next one in front of her, the next one to the next one and it goes until the message arrives to the first child in the line. She is responsible for collecting the balls. The child in front can take only one ball at a time then put it to the basket; each time you change the place of the basket so that the game is still challenging.

You may decide that children change their place after picking one ball or 3 balls, and the first one in the line goes to the end and becomes a guide, until all children take all roles. Finally, any group that collects more balls wins.

Your practice:

First of all, I highly recommend and actually encourage you to play these games with your adult friends and experience them for yourself before you introduce them to your students or group of kids you intend to work with.

Trust me, you'll learn so much about yourself by these games.

Then,

Sit by a friend and share about your experiences. Observe how much you can trust. Why do you trust some people easier and don't trust some others at all? What characteristics exist in others or in you that forms trust or mistrust?

How do you trust yourself to be a leader or a guide and take responsibility for another or a group of people?

In which area do you think you must work on to improve your trust and communication to other people?

9. Partner Yoga:

Definitely one of the excellent ways to get self-adjusted in yoga asanas is by the support of each other. When two kids do the asanas together, they are encouraged to take deep breaths and try to adjust their breathings to each other. If the partners listen to each other's breathings, they can help each other to adjust themselves with their breath in the posture. In this way flexibility can be increased as well.

When we practice stretching exercises together, we can:

- Stretch the body in a more fun and caring way.

- Balancing skills are practiced more.

- Move with the awareness that each of our movements affects the other one.

- It is better to constantly give feedback to each other and share the feelings you receive in each stretch or each exercise during the postures.

- Maintain and increase our communication with each other by using words, facial expressions, contact, breathing and even your thoughts.

- Develop trust and conversation.

- Give and receive safe pressure and contact.

- You get more intimate and close with your friends, family or child.

When you help each other in doing asanas, it is important to communicate with love and compassion. Be aware of how stretches affect your body. Observe, listen to your partner and how she feels while doing the exercise, and be careful not to hurt each other by putting excessive pressure.

Encourage children to ask the following questions from each other while doing the partner asanas:

- How do you feel?

- Is the pressure too much or you'd rather stretch more?

- Please let me know if either pressure or stretch is too much.

Here you'll be introduced to some partner yoga postures and how they can be done in collaboration. Of course know that there are so many varieties of postures that can be design and done in pairs, but here you'll get a taste of few asanas then to learn more start by playing with a friend and discover together amazing partner poses or find a partner yoga class and learn more variations and poses which can be done in pairs.

1-Uttanasana:

Ask kids to stay in pairs in front of each other.

Open the legs shoulder distance apart. opening the chest and straightening their backs.

Then stretch their arms and place them on each other's shoulders. Then bend forward, finding the right distance between them. They will bend from their hip joints as shown in the picture. By gently pushing each other's shoulders down and stretching their backs, they help each other to open their chests and adjust each other in the posture.

It's a nice stretch, helps for kids with scoliosis by lengthening the spine and finding more space in the vertebrates.

Variation in the posture:

-They can hold each other's hands, naturally there will be more distance between them.

-You can do the same variations with legs wide open in (Prasarita Padottanasana)

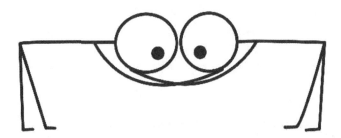

2-Some standing chest and shoulder openings:

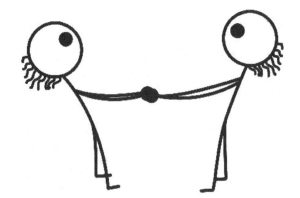

Standing in pairs facing each other, ask kids to find the right distance between them so that they can stretch their arms, while holding each other's hand and support each other while they're opening their chests.

looking up, opening the chest, arms are totally straight, hold each other's hand tightly, then release each one hand by stretching toward the back. Do this a few times by

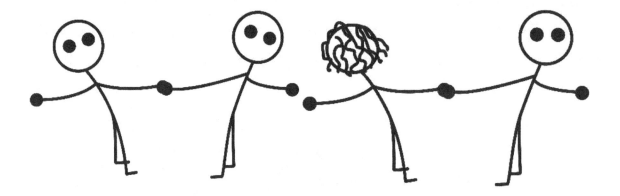

Changing hands. You can open up to the same side, then add a twist so that each one face the opposite side and adding a nice twist in the spine.

3-UtkatAsana:

a- Stand in front of each other in pairs. Hold each other's hands. then finding the right distance both, bend their knees and sit in utkatasana.

For adding variation, they can lean back, hold each other's hand tight so that they can support each other then release & stretch one hand back, opposite side of each other as shown in the picture below.

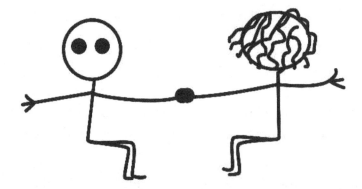

b- Stand back to back, clasp each other's elbows, then find the right distance and by leaning to each other's back sit in Utkatasana, like you are sitting in a chair.

Then to add some fun, a nice exercise is: one child will support the other while the other child pushes her back toward the back of her partner and slowly lifts his legs, while the other one slowly bent down.

They need to do the right balance while shifting one weight up. Supervise and assist each group for this partner posture.

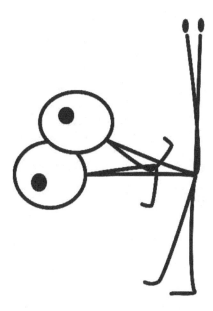

4-Vrikshasana:

Ask kids to stay in pairs next to each other. Shoulder to shoulder. The feet parallel to each other while standing will be the base.

They will stretch their arms which the shoulders are touching and put their palms together.

Then bending the opposite knee taking it up and with the other hand they will hold each other's ankle and support each other in the balancing posture. change sides and do the other leg.

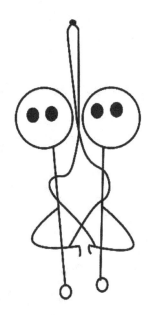

As a variation, they can position on opposite sides. Meaning one face the front, the other the back.

5-Padangusthasana

Another standing balancing posture. 2 kids will face each other, find the right distance. Then both lift their right legs up and with the help of the left hand place the foot in the opposite hip joint of their partner.

Once found the right balance, they will place one hand on each other's shoulder while opening the other arms. You can open the opposite arms and add a twist in the pose.

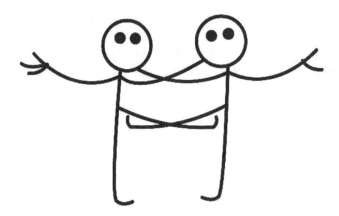

You can do this posture in groups of 3 and play with opening the same and opposite arms, while placing their same foot on each other's thighs as support.

Don't forget to change legs and do both sides.

6- Trikonasana and Parsvakonasana:

For doing these postures together, you'll ask 2 kids to go to the posture while having their backs supporting each other.

Back to back Trikonasana then Parsvakonasana. You can play by holding each other's knees, or ankles, or clasping hands while being in the pose.

They can also play with going through a flow of asanas. For example:

Standing with their legs wide apart, back to back they start by going to Trikonasana and follow the posture as bellow:

Trikonasana->Parsvakonasana->Ardha Chandrasana (Half moon)

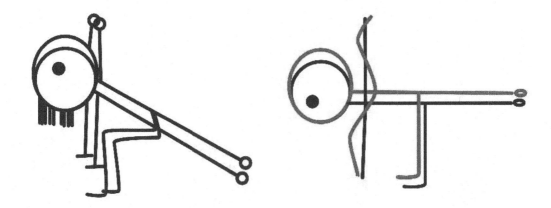

7-Virabhadrasana2:

The kids in a pair of 2, stand next to each other while having their feet 3 times shoulder distance apart. They will turn out the back foot of the one placed next to each other and point out the toes to the next foot. Ready to go to Virabhadrasana2.

Then they stretch one arm up and hold each other's hands with a gentle backbend, they also hold the other hands lower than the other and they can twist to one side then another by shifting their holding hands up & down in turn.

Then change the leg and do the other side.

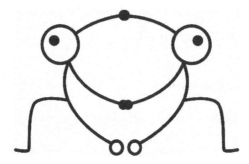

8-Janu Sirsasana

Ask kids to sit in dandasana while their feet are touching and they keep the sole of their feet together, Then they both bend their right knees and place the sole of their foot on their inner thigh. After, they will hold each other's hand, lean back at first then stretch their arms and bring their hands forward on each other's arms or shoulders depending on how far they can bend while keeping their back straight. Change sides.

Variations you can add:

Hold opposite hands then twist each to one side and then the other side.

They can also do the same variations in pastchimuttanasa and other varieties of Janu Sirsasana.

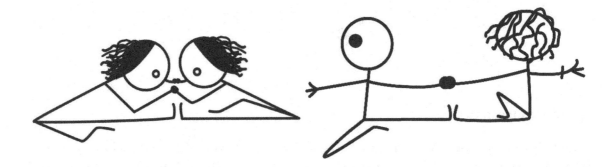

9- Upavishtakonasana:

Ask pairs of kids working together, to sit in front of each other with their legs wide open. Ask them to keep their knee caps facing upward, pointing the toes up and their feet touching.

Ask them to stretch their arms then hol each other's hands. And one by one then can bend forward by keeping their back straight and bending from the hip joints. One will bend the other will gently pushing her partner forward while she can lean back.

Aftcr both went to the forward bend. Then ask them to sit up straight and hold their right hands while each twist to one side and stretch the other hand. Change hands and twist to the other side.

You can cross the hands and play by twisting to different sides.

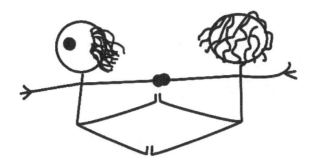

10-Navasna:

Children sit in front of each other, bend their knees and come forward until they can hold each other's hand. Then find the right space between each other. They will bring the sole of their feet join together keeping the feet together, slowly start by stretching the legs while having their back straight. If they can not completely straighten their back, tell them to not hunch their back, instead just stay with their knees bended.

Once they found their balance in the posture you can guide them into different variations:

-They can play by bending their knees while hands are still holding on to each other, then taking the legs under their arms and opening the legs looking up. Then again bend the knees and take them inside the hands. They can play a few times by bringing the legs in & out!

-They can also release opposite hands, stretch the arms and twist to different sides. Then change hands and twist to the other side. They can do the twist with both open and closed legs.

It's so much fun and one of my favorite partner poses! :)

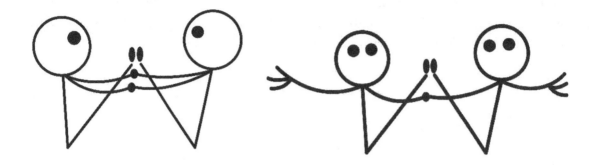

11- Virasana & backbend

Ask pairs of kids to sit back to back. Shoulder to shoulder. Then one is going to virasana while the other is gently pushing her back and goes to a back opening. They can clasp each other's hands. Then they can change sides.

One fun game here is:

While they are sitting back to back. Both bend their knees and place the sol of their foot down. They will clasp their elbows and with collaboration, counting to 3, they try to stand up without letting go of each other's arms.

Once they are up, they can play the balancing pose we learned here in variations on Utkatasana posture (number 3).

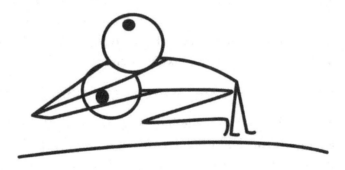

12-Adho Mukha svanasana & half arm balance:

You can start this partner pose using the wall and once they find enough confidence and balance in the pose they can do it without the support of the wall.

Ask one kid to stand with her heels up the wall and her toes down the earth and go to the downward dog.

You'll help the other kid to place her feet one by one on her partner's botox, while she is having her hands strongly rooter on the ground and her arms should be in such distance that when she goes up it her hips create a 90 degree shape with her upper body. You'll also find the 90degree measurement in her arms and upper body.

The child with her legs up to 90 degree will push her partner's hips up and toward the wall so that the one in downward dog feels her arms becoming weightless. Then she will be ready to shift her arms up like wings around her chest.

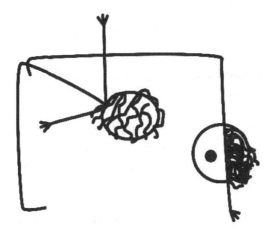

13- Dhanurasana

Ask one kid to lie on her belly, and bend her knees and flex her toes. The other kid will sit on the sole of her feet. Then the lying kid will take her hand back as if she will go to Dhanurasana posture, but instead of holding her own ankles, the other kid will hold her hands and gently push her back by leaning back herself.

This looks like a chariot and it's driver which you've also been introduced to in the asana and games section.

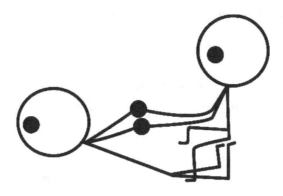

14- Ustrasana:

Ask kids in pairs to sit on their knees while having their back at each other and while tucking their toes under, join their heels together. Then slowly both will go to the camel posture. Bending gently backward with stretching their arms and keeping their belly button forward.

They can play by going backward to touch each other's hands then come back again and after a few rounds they can hold each other's hands and take a few breaths in the pose. If they feel uncomfort in their lower back they should immediately come back from the pose and go to child pose.

It's nice to do the partner virasana and other partner backbend poses we went through before in this section as a follow up to this practice.

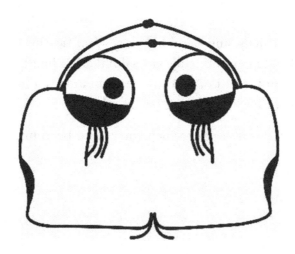

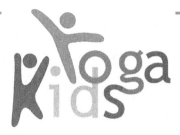

CHAPTER 14
Breathing Games and Exercises

In this section, we introduce games and exercises which have a significant role in making children aware of their breathing. Breath exercises Helps to balance emotions. By being aware of our breathing we would be able to eliminate our tension, calm the nervous system, heals depression and weariness.

The principle of breathing or Pranayama

Most people just use a part of the capacity of their respiratory system or lungs for breathing. People who have short breath and expand only a small part of the rib cage have bent shoulders, feel a painful pressure on top of their neck and back, and suffer from anoxia. They get tired easily and don't know why. With yoga respiratory exercises, in addition to preventing these issues, life energy (Prana) and health are guaranteed. The most important outcome of proper breathing is Pranayama or the subtle energy obtained from the vital breathing. Controlling Prana leads to mind control. The biggest sign of Prana in the body is the healthy movement of lungs. This movement operates like a wheel, and stimulates other body forces.

In normal breathing, we absorb just a little Prana, but when we concentrate and consciously regulate our breathing, we absorb a lot of Prana.

The four stages of breathing:

If we pay attention to our breathing, we find that a good breathing consists of four stages:

Inhalation, pause (holding the breath), exhalation, pause (with empty lungs). Inhalation represents the receiver, and says that the person tends to find a position for himself on the earth. When we inhale, we pull power and strength inside us. Pausing with air-filled lungs represents persistence. Exhalation is the symbol of "other" or our giving "self", and creates a feeling of liberation. Pausing with empty lungs represents silence and trust in the body and in everything.

Breathing Exercises in Children's Yoga Classes:

Children sometimes get restless in the class. If you start the class with respiratory exercises, you would find that these exercises have relaxing effects on children and enable them to have an active presence in the class. Some children get nervous when they have to speak in front of a crowd or in the class in front of other children, their neck and facial muscles get contracted and their breathing quickens, such that speaking becomes problematic to them. In such cases, deep breathing can help them and bring them peace and self-confidence. Respiratory exercises and chanting mantra help to cure children's stutter and respiratory problems, and also improves their concentration.

Exercises presented in this section, such as breathing exercises along with awareness and abdominal breathing, are very efficient in the class. You can do these exercises in sitting or lying down position. If you do exercises in a sitting position on a chair (for the schools), ask the children to completely put the soles of their feet on the ground and ask them to put their hands on their stomachs.

If the weather is good enough, you may let the window open while exercising, so that the children feel the open air flow.

Breathing Exercise 1
Observing & Recognizing our breath

Items needed: yoga mat

Our breathing takes place naturally, but we can master it. The first and most important step in this regard is feeling and observing our breath. Ask the children to lie on their mats in any position they are more comfortable, and stay still as long as they can. Then ask them if still any of their body parts are moving, or if any of their internal body organs are moving. If yes, which one? Children may notice that with every breath they take, their rib cage and abdomen go up and down. If they are lying on their stomachs, they may feel movement at their lumbar arch and pelvis with every breath they take. In such exercises, go to each of them, put your hand on the moving part of the body and say: "Very good, are you feeling the movement?" Explain to them that with every breath we take air flows into our lungs and the lungs inflate like a balloon, when we exhale, air comes out of the lungs, and the lungs deflate. Enlargement and shrinkage of the lungs cause the rib cage, abdomen and back to move up and down.

Different variations of the exercise:

In case of doing this exercise right after other exercises, the child feels her breathing more in the rib cage area, and can feel better her heart beat.

Ask the children to get into different lying positions like lying on the stomach, side or back, and each time ask them where in their body they felt the movement. This exercise can be done in a sitting or standing position too. In this mode, inhalation, exhalation and their movement in the body would be more tangible, and as a result, children should have more concentration.

Breathing Exercise 2
Abdominal breathing

Items needed: yoga mat.

Breathing takes place in us spontaneously but not all of us breathe efficiently and optimally.

Most of us are used to breathing improperly, for example breathing only from the chest.

By conscious breathing exercises we can lead the breath to the abdominal areas instead of the rib cage. When the stomach expands with each breath we take, it shows that the diaphragm is involved to fill the whole capacity of the lungs. You may do the breathing exercise 1 first, and then ask them to lie on their back and put their hands on their stomachs.

With each breath, ask them if they notice their abdominal ups and downs. This way you can guide them to the abdominal breathing.

With each inhalation, the abdomen fills with air, while with each exhalation, air escapes from the abdomen and the abdomen shrinks. Tell them that they should not do the exercise with pressure, and in fact the lungs should move the abdomen from inside. After the exercise, ask the children about their feelings during the respiratory exercises.

Different variations of the exercise:

While exercising, we usually breathe fast from the rib cage. You may first create fast breathing in children by some cardio practices, and then take them into abdominal breathing. This way, the shift in breathing from the rib cage to the abdomen would be more understandable to them.

Breathing Exercise 3
Blowing

Items needed: one leaf, cotton ball or a small piece of paper for each player.

With this entertaining game, we teach children how to control their breath by a deep, gentle blow. Ask the children to sit in a circle and give each of them the item you prepared, I will refer to a leaf for the ongoing explanation of the game.

They must put the leaf on the palm of their hands and blow it. Ask them: "What happens in your body when you blow?"

Then ask the children to repeat the game but this time, blowing stronger. Ask them how they felt it was different from the previous time. Ask them to blow the leaf with different pressures. Then ask them about the capacity of their own breath at different speed, while blowing the leaf.

Other variations of the exercise:

-Ask them to stand up and blow the leaf while standing.

-Ask them to lie on their bellies and blow the leaf in this position.

Then talk about the differences and in which form their breath had more capacity to blow the leaf.

Breathing Exercise 4
Witness the motion of breath

Items needed: A cotton ball and a straw for each child.

This exercise helps children to get to know their breathing better. Ask children to sit in a circle, and give each of them a cotton ball. Ask them to hold the cotton balls on their palms under their nose, and focus on it. Ask them: "What do you see? Try to naturally breathe through your nose; do you see the movement of the cotton ball with the rhythm of your inhalation and exhalation?"

Other variations of the exercise:

*Ask the children to repeat the exercise but this time breathe through their mouths.

*Ask them to yawn and look at the movement of the cotton ball in their hand.

*You may practice this breathing exercise after doing some fast yoga movements such as a few turns of the sun salutation. This way, children understand the difference between a normal breath and a fast breathing.

*Ask the children to lie on their bellies while staying in the circle facing each other. give each of them a straw (**To respect the ecosystem and also to promote the mentality of Limiting the use of plastic to protect our planet, use bamboo or organically paper made straws**). Blow the cotton ball on the ground with the help of the straw. You can consider a small circle in the middle of the circle so that kids aim the centre while blowing their cotton balls.

Breathing Exercise 5
Sounds

Playing this game, children understand the vibration of their body parts like head, throat and chest while making sounds. This exercise also strengthens the abdominal muscles and improves their respiratory capacity.

Ask kids to sit in a circle. Then guide them to open their mouth and as if they were yawning make a sound coming from their throat. This exercise helps to open the larynx, also known as the voice box. They open in order to help you to breath. When you pronounce the sounds in a vibrating mode, like chanting om mantra, air passes through the larynx causing the vocal cords to vibrate and produce sounds.

Now You are going to use different sounds which helps to deepen the breath.

"Breathe gently from your abdomen. We want to repeat the "Mmmm..." sound, with a loud and harmonious tone. repeated "Mmmm" sound, has a very affective vibration, since by making it you feel that the lips gently meet each other, and a special vibration occurs." You yourself always demonstrate the sound first so that the children are not shy to try. Usually when we make this sound together, a very pleasant vibration is created. You may practice this exercise with different letters of the alphabet.

You can follow up by asking these questions after they created the sound vibration in their circle:

When you chant the "M" sound, in which parts of your body do you feel vibration? You may repeat this question after collectively making "N", R, D, Z". How do your lips and tongue move when you make "B" sound? You may repeat the same question after collectively making "D, F, L, B, T, S, V" sounds.

What happens in your mouth while making "CH" sound? You may repeat the same question after collectively making "J, H, K, J, R, SH" sounds. In which of these sounds does your mouth open more widely?, "E, A, O"?

And this way you can play with different alphabetical letters and create different vibrations that also deepen the breath.

Other variations of this exercise:

-You may ask children to do this exercise in standing or even walking position.

-Ask them to hold their ears while making the sounds so that they can concentrate on the sound vibration inside their head. One of the sounds which can act like a mantra is "m". Ask them to hold their ears and make "mmmmm" sound (like a bee), repeat it with "zzzzzz" in which lips open slightly.

- Ask them to chant each other's names like a mantra by extending their favorite sounds in a loud voice, in a way which the breathing and sound comes from the abdomen and reaches to the upper body.

Breathing Exercise 6
Back-to-Back Breathing

Children should sit back to back. Ask them to breathe deeply and feel each other's breaths. When they inhale, they should let their back open and expand, as if the spine is getting longer by finding more space to breathe in between vertebrates. When exhaling, they should allow their body to release and relax without hunching in the back.

Breathing Exercise 7
Animal Breathing

1. Rabbit breathing: Three fast and deep breaths followed by a series of fast exhales through the nose. (Like KapalaBhati, Krya exercise) This is rabbit breathing for children. For making it more interesting for kids, you can tell them to scrunch up their noses while breathing or do it during the Rabbit posture.

2. Lion breathing: Sit on your knees and heels. If you feel any pressure on your knees, better to sit on a bolster with separated knees. put your hands on the knees, with your fingers wide open, like the lion claws. Open your chest, straighten your spine, Take a deep inhale and as you are exhaling open your mouth widely, Stick your tongue out, look up and exhale with a sound as a lion roars. Repeat it a few times, then go to child pose and rest.

3. Dog breathing: You can do this breathing exercise being in downward or upward dog. Stick out the tongue and breath out fastly through the mouth. If you look at dogs you'll see them breath like that, especially in hot seasons as it helps them to cool down.

4. Bee breathing (Brahmari): This is an ancient yogic breathing practices.Sit with your back straight and open your chest, cover your ears with your thumb and you can hold the other fingers on your head. Another form is to cover your ears with your thumbs then bring the other fingers on your face so that they are positioned above your eyebrows, on your eyes, around your lips and chin, then inhale through the nose, With close lips, whisper the repeating "mmmmmmmmmm" sound coming from the back of your throat, throughout your deep exhale. It vibrates like the sound of a bee in your head. Repeat the exercise 3 to 5 rounds.

5. Snake breathing (Shittali and Sitkari): This exercise is also an ancient yogic breathing practice. They both have cooling effects and it's very suitable in hot weathers to cool down the body's temperature.

Sit with your back straight and open your chest. Roll your tongue in your mouth while having your mouth slightly open. Some kids might not be able to roll their tongue. Tell such children to stick the tongue to the back of their mouth. Then take a deep breath in through your mouth and feel the cool air coming in through your inhale.

Then exhale through your nose. Close your eyes and do the practice for a couple of rounds.

Another way of this breathing practice is to open your mouth as if you are smiling while gently pressing your lower and upper teeth together. inhale deeply and gently through your teeth with a hissing sound. Feel the cool breath coming through your teeth. Then exhale through your nose.

6. Dragon breathing / Sun or Fire breathing (Kapalabhati): This is also an ancient yogi method of Krya (cleansing) helps cleaning the lungs and the respiratory tract, strengthens the abdominal muscles and refreshes the body with lots of oxygen and energy. Sit with your back straight, open your chest and inhale deeply through the nose. Then keep exhaling in a fast paste continuously and slow the rhythm as you end the last exhales, then breath deeply in and out for 3 rounds and go on for another 3 to 5 rounds of the "Dragon breath". Smaller children can gently do this exercise in animal games. To make it more interesting, you may do this exercise in other positions like the Fish pose.

Breathing Exercise 8:
Cloud and Angel Breathing

Cloud: lie down on your back and imagine you are a big, white, puffy, soft and peaceful cloud. Breathe in and exhale as deep as you can. Each time you breathe deeply in, imagine your cloud getting bigger and lighter and taking you higher in the blue sky. You may also use a magical carpet instead of a cloud, if it can relate to your class theme.

Angel: Sit with your back straight. Put the hands on the sides. Inhale and take the hands up like an angel's wings. Exhale and bring the hands back to the body sides. As you open your arms, breath in deeply, imagine your angel wings open up toward the sky. as you bring your arms down breathe out slowly and repeat the motion for a few times as an angel flying and spreading her sparkles into the earth. You may do this exercise either sitting or standing.

Breathing Exercise 9:
Self hug

Inhale and completely open the arms to the sides. Exhale and hug yourself tight. Put your hands on the opposite shoulders. Repeat it as many times as you want.

To make it more fun:

- Rock gently from side to side whilst hugging, or
- Pat the body and make a wish for yourself (or another loved one) for a great day!

Breathing Exercise 10:
Counting the Breaths

Ask children to sit in a crossed leg position with their back straight then, Guide them as follows:

Bring one hand up next to your ear. Lift one finger at a time as you breathe in through your nose and count in your mind: 1, 2, 3, 4, 5. (count out loud for them). Pause for a second with your hand up. Slowly breathe out through your nose, counting backwards 5, 4, 3, 2, 1, and lowering a finger at a time for each number. Your hand is now making a feast. repeat for 3 to 5 times.

Breathing Exercise 11:
Straw and Cotton Breathing

Items needed: straw (**To respect the ecosystem and also to promote the mentality of Limiting the use of plastic to protect our planet, use bamboo or organically paper made straws**), cotton ball.

All children sit in a circle. Give each child a straw. You are going to start by keeping a cotton ball in the palm of one hand and by a deep inhale through the straw, the cotton ball will stick to the straw. You need to hold the inhale to pass the cotton ball to the one next to you. She will take a deep inhale and collect the cotton ball with her straw and pass it to the other one next to her. This goes on until it reaches the end of the circle.

This is an interesting and joyful exercise, while at the same time increases the respiratory capacity and deepens breathing.

A fun team game:

Kids can form 2 groups. They will lie on their bellies, each team opposite to the other. You can draw a line in front of each group which means the entrance of their gate. Then you distribute some cotton balls in the middle of the field. kids are all holding a straw in their mouth. When you announce the starting of the game, they all start by blowing into the straw and driving the cotton balls into the opposite group. Each team tries to prevent the cotton balls from entering the gate and crossing the line. Once the cotton ball reaches the line, You'll leave it there. At the end of the game, when you announce the time out, the team with the least cotton balls in their gate wins.

> ***Attention: In order to practice these games, make sure that the floor is properly cleaned and disinfected, otherwise, Don't introduce the practice.**

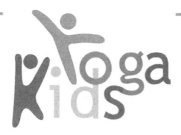

CHAPTER 15
Inviting to Silence games

Sometimes the class falls apart and becomes disorganized. Children chat constantly, jump around, scream and move the equipment in the classroom. You may almost feel that you are incapable of controlling the class. In such situations, don't panic! don't shout and lose control! take a deep breath and you can use these amazing games & ideas we will go through in this chapter to invite kids into silence without even mentioning that you want them to calm down! It's like magic tricks and by using these games they will be invited to stay in silence in a fun way which satisfies their curious nature as well as transmitting the message of silence. Children will sit in silence without being forced to, and eagerly will pay attention to you. You have to know that a kids yoga class is not going to be silent all the time and you have to expect and accept their enthusiasm knowing that Sometimes class goes on with play and laughter which is totally fine, keep calm and accept & enjoy their energy level as it is; you should be flexible in your way of thinking with children. Just do your best to introduce the practices in a way that they can understand and invite them to cooperate without ever pushing them into doing anything by force.

These games in this chapter also help children to sit in silence, close their eyes for some seconds and look within themselves. In fact, this is an opportunity for preparing children to sit in meditation.

Now, let's go through some of these games:

The telephone game:

You may have experienced this game as a child. I encourage you as I mentioned before to first experience and play these games with your adult friends then introduce it to children.

The game is as follows:

All children sit in a circle. You might start by whispering a sanskrit name of an asana gently in the ear of the child in your right. She will transmit the message to the next one and the message keeps on delivering until it gets back to you!

Often, the word reaches back to you with a lot of changes, and creates a funny word or sentence making you all laugh and have fun.

Now someone else can start and repeat the game.

For smaller kids you better not use the asana names but a more simple word.

You can also use sentences.

While the message is passin, all kids are attentive and in silence in order to hear the words and wait eagerly to hear the outcome.

The silent Buddhas:

Ask the children to sit in a circle with closed eyes. Tell them that they are all silent Buddhas in meditation. describe the qualities of a Buddha in meditation: He is silent, sits with a straight spine, has gentle smiles and does not open his eyes while he breathes deeply and silently.

You can first start the Game yourself by holding a bell or a Tibetan bowl. You'll go around and you'll tell them you are going to choose a perfect silent buddha and ring the bell slowly next to her ear. You might wait a bit while encouraging them to stay still while keeping their eyes closed and You might also add that they all look like perfect Buddha statues but you have to choose one to start the game. Then choose a child, ring the bell and take her place to sit. Then she will continue by choosing another child in the circle as follows. You might conduct the game yourself by pointing out to the kids who have not yet been chosen, in order for all the kids to have their turn on going around the circle holding the bell.

By the end You can invite them to open their eyes and they'll notice that everyone has changed their starting sitting place!

Variety of the game:

-The silent Buddha and the trouble maker:

This is a partner game in which the two children sit facing each other. One is a silent Buddha, who sits in meditation, with a straight back and a beautiful smile on her face.

The second one becomes the intruder who will try to break the silence of the buddha by distracting her. She can make funny gestures to make her laugh, telling her appropriate funny jokes, but she can't touch the Buddha at all or use any kind of violent words or actions (you should be very strict about this rule in the game, to keep them safe). The Buddha will resist the intruder and keep her peaceful state as much as she can, once she starts laughing or coming out of the meditative pose, they'll wait for the bell by sitting both quietly. You'll keep time and when you announce the end of one round, they will change roles.

Cards:

Items needed: playing cards with pictures of animals – yoga mat.

Ask the children to sit in a circle and close their eyes. Put a card under each mat. Now ask them to open their eyes and look at the picture on the card without letting anyone see it. Then one child says 3 characteristics of the animal whose picture is on her card. The rest must guess what animal is that.

It is suggested that you use cards which might have some information about the animal or species you want them to talk about. You can also make these cards yourself and gather some facts about the related creature and put it on one side of the cards so that kids have the option to read about the related animal they want others to guess.

Anyone who guesses right has to go to the yoga posture of that animal and the others should copy her. Then they will change their sitting space and we continue the game until all cards have been revealed.

Other variations of the game:

- You can sometimes use this method to choose a partner randomly by putting similar cards in pairs under their mats. The two having the same cards become partners in the subject you want to guide them into.

- Instead of explaining and stating 3 points about the animal, ask the children to make the shape of that animal with yoga asanas, through pantomime showing the reactions of it and making silent movements; the rest should guess the animal's name.

- When everyone is sitting in a circle with closed eyes, and you are guiding them to sit in silence, quietly & secretly put a card under one chosen child. Do it the way nobody realizes where the card is. distract them by pretending to put the card on a few mats, then once you really chose a child, Slowly touch her shoulder as a sign; She knows just by the sign you indicated to her, that she has the card. Explain to the children in advance that whoever has the card under their mat should be neutral and act in a way that no one will understand she is the one with the card under her mat! Now ask the children to open their eyes and guess who has the card.

After the intended person is found, she looks at the picture of the card without letting anyone see it and points out three characteristics of it. This picture could be a fruit, an animal with a related asana or anything else. The other children will guess what the secret card is, then once revealed, they 'll all go to the pose with their bodies.

Walking with the Bell:

Items needed: Some bells.

Divide children to groups of two. One child of each group stands on one side of the classroom next to the members of the other groups, and her teammates stand on the other side in front of her with bells in hand. The game must be played in complete silence. The child who has the bell in hand should move toward the one in front of her so quietly and concentrated that not a slightest sound comes out of the bell. If there is a slightest sound, the child has to get back to the first point and start walking again. When she succeeds in reaching the opposite child, they change their place and she gives the bell to her teammate. The aim is that both team members reach each other so concentrated that the bell stays silent during their walk.

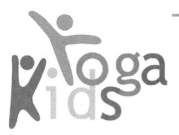

CHAPTER 16
Sitting in Meditation and Observing Different Senses

Meditation means to observe the thoughts and to stay in a state where body and mind are completely liberated; or in other words, it means to be in the present moment. This is much more natural for the children to be at the moment, in comparison to the adults, because they don't carry so many thoughts with them and their minds are not involved in different judgments about themselves and others.

Meditation exercises help the children to experience more peace, get concentrated and also helps them to understand their feelings. These exercises help them get themselves better. Always encourage children to express their feelings after a guided meditation, and be aware of their thoughts. If you see a problem, take a note, so that you work on this particular problem the next session. In these exercises, first ask the children to sit in a crossed leg position. First, tell them the three following rules:

1- The spine should be straight and stretched toward the ceiling (like a flower grown toward the sun).
2- Open your inner smile(open the chest). Open your Upper Smile (on the lips).
3- Be aware of your breath and the gentle air passing under your nostrils.

You can start by asking them to first close their eyes then bring one hand under their nostrils and feel the air passing through. Then make them conscious of their sitting position and once ready you can take them into a short guided visualization into your chosen subject related to the theme of your class.

You can choose different emotions from positive to negative such as (sitting in happiness, bully, anger, fear, friendship, beauty, happiness and...) so that children know that it is ok for them to feel different emotions and you give them the right solutions on how to deal with them.

For example, sitting in the sense of bullying gives them the experience that if they have ever bullied someone, what kind of feeling have they caused in them. Always remember to ask them, at the end of such exercises, to put forward their experience. If a child confesses that she has formerly bullied another child, you should never blame or shame her; just without any judgment ask her to express her feelings and then explain the feeling and give them a solution so that next time they encounter such feelings they'll know how to deal with it. For example in our bullying example mentioned above you can tell them: "First of all I want to applaud you for having the courage to admit about your action. Sometimes we do or say things that we don't really mean, But It can hurt somebody's feelings and we don't want to promote any bad feelings in anyone as we now know how hurtful it can be. But You can always apologize if you realized you've done or said something wrong and next time you want to say something just think what might the other person feel and don't say anything that can be hurtful, instead just express how you really feel."

Or if you see some emotion like anger arises in them, guide them into releasing anger solutions you'll learn in this chapter and always talk about the emotions, the effects they can transmit and the better solution to deal with it.

Make a space in such that all kids feel welcome in it with any kind of emotion they have. They must feel that they are accepted in your class unconditionally so that they can trust you and express their emotions; they must not think they are judged. They should not be afraid of being punished or questioned, or feel guilty, because these kinds of feelings would not necessarily lead to a change in their behavior. They should feel safe enough to be who they are and know that they are understood and if you build such a relationship with kids, they will respect you and mostly listen to what you say.

You must show them that they can make mistakes, and it's totally ok but we learn from it and move on. They will know that you are a grown up friend they can count on and trust without being threatened, judged or criticized all the time. If they feel understood and loved, they will coope with you.

All of these exercises can be done in school classes, and these hints may help to solve the problems they might have with their classmates.

When you want to start the beginning meditation, and invite them to their circle, It's better that you first sit with them to begin, then once they have closed their eyes, stand up and walk around so that your attention is distributed among them evenly.

Sometimes you need to make them aware either with a slight tap on their bodies or by pouring an imaginary magical powder or by pointing with eyes or by looking, encourage them to keep their eyes closed. These guided visualizations should be short and completely clear, and expressed in a simple and understandable language.

In the guided meditation, once a feeling is introduced, I always like to ask children to give a color to the feeling and ask them about it at the end of the meditation in their sharing circle. Colors have different meanings and different effects into our lives. I'll go through that later in the related chapter about "the colors and their effects". But here I might not mention the color in all meditations but you can always add it into your designed session.

1- Sitting Still

Ask kids to sit on a yoga pillow or short block in one of the sitting postures. Putting something under their bottom helps them to keep their back straight. Ask them to put their hands on their thighs above the knees, Keeping their palms up, connecting the thumb and index finger together. Explain to them that in fact by connecting index finger and thumb, they can connect to their inner self and by having the under finger toward the sky, they are announcing to the universe that they are ready to receive all that the gifts life has to offer them. Then prepare them for meditation in the following order:

*"First be aware of your contact with the grounds while sitting. Feel that you have roots in the ground, and at the same time, you are connected to the sky and grow toward the sun. Breathe regularly and watch which parts of your body move while breathing. Watch your thoughts like a series of clouds passing by in the blue sky, feel that your breath is the wind and with each breath you take, set aside a piece of cloud, and ultimately imagine the very blue sky. If there is still a thought (cloud), don't judge it; good, bad, right, wrong, just look at it as it is.

*Don't stay with any passing thoughts. Just look and let them like suspended clouds pass through the sky of your mind so that you can see the clearly beautiful, clear blue sky."

*Let children sit in this position between 5 to 10 minutes, depending on their age & condition, then gently ask them to open their eyes, share about their experience one by one and express whatever crossed their minds during the meditation.

2-Sitting in Friendship

Children can form their friendships from early ages. Childhood friendship may end up in a break time in the school yard or may remain a lifetime.

Children can learn the value of friendships through playing.

*Ask the children to sit quietly and close their eyes, same as what they did in the first exercise of this section, and guide them as follows:

"As you are sitting with your closed eyes, try to just look at your thoughts and how they just come and go in your mind. You probably have a friend or there is someone you love deeply in your life. I want you to think about that friend. What is so good about that particular person which comes first into your mind? What characteristics does a good friend have in your opinion? If you were to give a color to the feeling of remembering a true friend, what would that color be? What is the color of friendship in your opinion? Do you think you are a good friend for your own friends?"

*Ask children to remain with the sense of friendship for some time, then ask them to gently open their eyes. Then you can talk a little about friendship as follows:

"There are so many things you can do when you have good friends. You can laugh, play and speak with your friends. You can help each other and give the gift of hope and smile to each other when you feel sad. Sometimes you may also not agree with your friend and that might end up in some issues in your friendship. Maybe you and your friend would not like to play the same game. Maybe sometimes you tell or do something and hurt each other's feelings. That happens sometimes too.

When you have a problem with your friends, It's a great idea to talk to each other; try to be honest and share your real emotions with them. Together you may come to a solution or if your problem is not solved, you can get help from an adult whom you trust. But friendships are important and it's better that you take good care of each other so that together you can overcome many problems when they accrue in any forms but also to have lots of fun with each other"

Then let them share their thoughts, experiences and ask each one of them what was the color of friendship for them in their guided meditation.

3-Sitting in the teasing feeling (bullying)

A very common - and bad habit- between kids, is to mock each other. Sometimes this happens through physical contact, sometimes the "ought teasing", such as name calling, regardless of the possible pain caused. Unfortunately, it happens in schools a lot, it's nice to pay attention to it and try to solve it.

Ask the kids to sit down with their eyes closed, return to the first exercise. And tell them:

"Observe your thoughts just the way they are. Sometimes you might bother your friends by mocking them, kicking them, pushing them or calling them names, and they might have been upset with you. Or even you might have been upset with your friends, who have annoyed you or called you names. What have you felt when you were annoyed with another child? Or when you were annoying some children?

Let them stay with their emotions for a few minutes, then ask them to open their eyes and discuss their thoughts. The best way is for you to stay as neutral as possible so that the children find the courage to speak openly and dare to show their real emotions. Then you can bring the topic up in this order:

"Have you ever told the person who's troubled you or has made fun of you how bad you felt inside?"

"Try to express your emotions next time when it happens to you, and observe carefully, if you feel that you've done the same thing to someone else and you've felt bad inside, you might go to that person and say that you're sorry, then try to not do it again. If you feel shy and embarrassed to talk to the person face-to-face, say it inside of yourself, and promise yourself never to repeat it.

4- Sitting in Beauty

Children learn very quickly to compare what they are and what they have with others; big, bigger, biggest, good, better, best, beautiful, more beautiful, most beautiful.

"I am the biggest; I want to be the best; mine is the best; yours is ugly."

These are the conversations they make with each other.

Self-confidence comes from inside. So does beauty. This exercise helps the children to understand they don't have to compare themselves with others, since everyone has their own beauty and that they are all perfect as they are.

*Ask the children to sit with closed eyes (exercise 1); then guide them as follows:

"Try to sit gently and watch your thoughts. You are beautiful. Your clothes don't make you beautiful or ugly. You are not more beautiful than others. Maybe you are beautiful in a different way, but this is not important. What is important is that you yourself know that you are beautiful both from inside and outside. Each person has their own beauty and no one can be compared to another, just look at nature. All flowers are beautiful but we just prefer and choose different flowers due to our own sense of beauty but no one can say a flower is more beautiful than another. It's just a personal taste. In the same way people are also different and no one can define what a real beauty is, the only thing we all know is that, when a person has a kind heart, no mater what they look like they are the most beautiful people in the world as the gift of a kind heart makes people shine from outside with their big inner light. Do you know any person like that? If you do you are a very lucky person. You can also be that person yourself!"

Then, after a while ask them to open their eyes and share their feelings with each other.

5- Sitting in Happiness

Children can learn from an early age to be happy and grateful for what they have in life.

Being happy has direct contact with trust and self-confidence. Happiness and joy also is expressed by physical signs in our body and there are different ways we react to it.

Being aware of these emotions and paying attention to the physical changes give kids the awareness to recognize the feeling and the effects they have in their lives and make them choose more wisely about the way they express their emotions.

*Ask the children to sit in a circle with closed eyes (exercise 1):

"Imagine yourself being very happy! Remember an event that made you so happy lately. How do you feel when you remember that pleasant memory? Do you feel happy? Where do you feel the happiness most in your body? Put your hands in that area of your body, you feel the happiness more? What color does have that happy feeling for you? Show me now your best happiness expression! How do you feel now?"

Let children remain in this state for a few moments, and then ask them to open their eyes and talk about their experience.

6-Sitting in Anger

Anger makes tension and contraction in the body. If someone is angry and doesn't find a way to express it, she gets muscle contraction, and this may lead to future physical problems. Anger releasing techniques may greatly solve our problems. To make this more clear, we should first teach children to get to know their emotions.

Ask children to sit in a comfortable position, close their eyes (exercise 1), and guide them as follows:

"Sit silently with your eyes closed and try not to think about anything; just watch those things which at this moment go through your mind. Do you feel angry sometimes? What makes you so angry? What color is anger? In which part of your body you feel anger?"

We should not prolong this part of the practice while they have their eyes closed, because the goal of this exercise is to recognize the feeling of anger not creating it. Children need just a few short moments to observe the anger inside them and its external reflection in their body. After they open their eyes, ask them in which part of their body they felt anger, and then present some solutions for releasing the internal anger that is piled up in that part of their body.

For example, if they feel anger in their feet, they can jump up and down, stamp with their feet; If they felt it in their hands then hit the pillow with their hands or punch in the air. If they feel anger in their throat, they can shout if the atmosphere of the class is protected and you are not disturbing any neighbors, otherwise they can do the Lion posture (Simhasana) and remove the anger from their throats.

After knowing about their anger and getting to know this sensation better, offer them some solutions to release their anger and switch it with peace and happiness.

What is important is to make them understand that anger is natural. It's the way they react to the anger that's very important.

It's natural to get angry sometimes, and they can express their anger in a way which is not harmful to anyone.

Recommended ideas to release anger:

1. Lion (Simhasana)
2. Volcano: Ask the children to go into Mountain position and stand as a mountain. They should imagine that they've become a volcano mountain. Then they outflow any senses that they want to release out of the volcano. While doing it they open their legs and bring their hands over their heads and then they go back to the first position.
3. Tarzan: Ask them to make a sound like Tarzan and hit their chests with their hands, like tarzan.
4. Funny monkeys: Everyone on the ground with their knees bent and their hands on the top of their heads, do the monkey voice. "Ha ha Hoo hoo ha ha..."
5- Balloon:

   First form: Ask them to stand and bloat themselves like a balloon. Then they imagine a needle popping the balloon and it exploding suddenly.

   Second form: Ask them to stand and bloat themselves like a balloon. Imagine that the balloon is released and all the air empties out slowly and the balloon falls to the ground.

   Third form: Bloat the colourful and small balloons and spread them around, then ask the children to walk on them and make them explode.

   Fourth form – bloat a series of balloons and release them in the air. It's better to ask kids help, to bloat the balloons. Then invite them to explode the balloons in the air.

6. Jelly: each child imagines themself as a colourful jelly, and shakes their body with a noise from inside.
7. Untying the knots: they feel like there are knots all around their bodies; they untie all these knots from top to bottom and get free.
8. Speaking Gibberish: expressing words and anger by making meaningless sounds. In this method, the energy of anger vents without anyone being insulted. Meanwhile, it causes laughter and calms the angry person.
9. Punching to the pillow or in the air.
10. Biting apples.

11. Becoming popcorn: ask the children to imagine they have turned into corn seeds and gather their hands and feet in sitting position. Then they start to jump up & down like corn seeds becoming popcorns.
12. Stumbling on the ground.
13. Tapping on the legs with my hand.
14. Tornado: they constantly spin for a while, along with their anger, and suddenly release themselves on the mat.
15. Woodcutter movement: You can either imagine cutting the woods in the air or you can use bolsters as trund and they can hit the bolster.

7- Sitting in Fear

Just like anger, fear is also a completely natural emotion which should be understood. To start this exercise and for the children to feel safe to express their fear, you had better start with yourself as an example and say: "I also have some fears. For example I am afraid of darkness", then present your solutions for dealing with this emotion.

Again as we already experienced with anger, we stay for a short time just for kids to recognize their fear but we don't want to provoke them into feeling scared.

You can instruct them in this manner:

Invite them to close their eyes and stay for a while with the sense of fear. Ask them where they feel the fear and what is their body reaction to this feeling. What color has fear for them? After a while, ask them to open their eyes and put their hands under their belly buttons. Explain to them about their powers and their inner light. Tell them whenever they're scared of something, remember that there is a light in their inner selves which destroys all the darkness around them. Then ask them to raise their right hand up and put their left hand over their belly button (solar plexus.) With every deep inhale they get power from the sun and by giving out the sound Ha! they express their powers. Then you can use some injunctive sentences like the examples given below to make them feel powerful and confident.

"I'm full of power."

"I use my power in the way of peace and helping others."

"When I feel sad, I look for the sun."

"When I feel scared, I look for my inner light."

We can use the seed meditation as well, to help them face their fears with courage and to hold their powers.

-The Seed Meditation:

Ask the children to go into the Mouse pose and guide them as follows: "Imagine that you are some seeds planted in the ground. First, all is dark around you, then sunlight shines on you. Slowly you start to grow and burst out from the ground." Then start to build the image of the seed waking up and growing towards the sun.Becoming a beautiful flower. Make it fun by singing a nice related poem (as example below) or playing nice and happy music.

Seed song:

I am a little seed!!
I am a colorful seed!
Tiny, round and small I am!
planted in the earth I am!
In the dark, hidden I am!
Out comes the sun, happy and shiny sun!
Down comes the rain, soft and suiting rain!
Here I grow!
Grow, Grow Grow!
And Here I come!
Happy & sound!
A beautiful flower, kissing the sun!

You can use the same idea or other ideas you come up with in the related subject, facing kids fears during your sessions.

For example, if they are afraid of the sea and ocean in water-related games, You can guide them into visualizing a protective bubble of light around them or the company of an imaginary dolphin friend...Or if they are afraid of an animal, you want to take them into the posture, You can use your imaginary magic power or any other tools to make them feel safe and protected. Especially in younger kids.

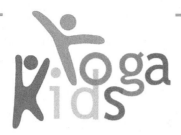

CHAPTER 17
Relaxation or Savasana

Here, I will take you into some short yoga Nidra or relaxing guided meditations for ending the yoga session with. It's the savasana part of yoga for kids.

Some guided imaginations are mentioned which help kids to relax and leave the class with a sense of peace and calmness.

At the end of your yoga activity, when children have been learning about asanas, played fun and entertaining games and used their energies during the whole practice, the last 5-10 minutes of your class, is one of the most impactful times of your session. Just like in adults yoga class, Savasana in the time you'll get the most and absorb the real essence of your yoga practice, in yoga kids session the way you end your session reflects their whole practice and helps them to restore and retain all that they learned in their yoga class.

Sometimes you can just guide them into a simple relaxation & body awareness like the few samples we have in this section, but most of the time we will use an ending story to make our session more pleasant and fruitful.

We all love stories. Many sages, sufi & zen masters used stories to come to a point. Also we can find so many interesting stories on sages of India, Deities, God and Goddesses in indian methodology also there are amazing stories behind most of the asanas.

One of the most powerful magic we possess in this life is our power of imagination.

Today we know how we can manifest our dreams by using our power of imagination. Children have a very creative mind and they can easily imagine and create a phantasy world in their minds. Now, imagine using this power of imagination since childhood to manifest our wishes and take total control over our destiny!

"A beautiful mind creates a beautiful world"

When kids picture peace, love, unity & all the constructive qualities in their mind, they are drawing a future map for their lives. They become compassionate human beings who love and respect their earth and all its creatures.

In this short time kids lie down and close their eyes, you can take them into a colorful world of possibilities and in the outcome they come out of the journey, refreshed, hopeful, brave and peaceful.

In order to be able to create such an effective guided visualization for kids, you need to feel your story, believe in it and tell the story from your heart.

Once you know your class theme, There are few important points you can use so that your story can be more impactful and effective. I will take you so few of these points:

1- Your voice:

The tone of your voice is very important. It shouldn't be so slow that kids can not hear you, or so loud that they'll be distracted. You should play with your tone, start by a suiting, calming tone to put them into a state of relaxation. Then sometimes raise your tone to make them alert also so that they don't fall asleep. you can then sometimes talk in a very slow tone as a whisper, like sharing a secret to attract their attention to listen to what you're saying.

2-Smile:

Yes! Your beautiful smile is needed in all areas! Even if people don't see you, your smile is reflected through your voice! Try it for yourself. Talk to a friend on your phone, or ask them to close their eyes, talk without your smile, then put a beautiful smile on your face and see how it changes everything! Even while reading this book, let's say right now! Shine that smile on your beautiful face, then continue! You instantly boost your creativity!

"Creativity is nurtured by your positivity"

2-Breath:

in between your story, remind them to breathe, and when you want to ask them to come back, guide them to count their breath and become conscious of their breathing before they sit up in their ending circle..

3- The story:

Use a story related to your class theme. The story should come to a point. It's not just a phantasy world you want to take them to, it's an imaginary land in which you remind them of all that they learned in their yoga session and what you want them to take out. For example if your theme was the ocean, by choosing a dolphin friend, you are reminding them to face their fears feeling guided and supported. Or when they reach the ocean to find the precious pearl, They will take a message out of the ocean of (love, courage, peace...) to share it as a secret into the world. And similar to that in different themes you can create a beautiful, attractive short story adding positive points and reminders of the qualities they can add as values in their lives.

4-Surprise gift:

Sometimes you'll need to promise them a surprise gift at the end of their guided meditation in order to invite them to lie down and stay in a relaxing position. The surprise gift can be as simple as a small flower, a little sticker with a note...

*Don't use that trick all the time so that it become an expectation, but maybe once a month if you find some positive points you can reward them with a little gift, it would encourage them and motivate them to respect the class rules and cooperate together to receive a reward when it is deserved and they'll know it.

5- Distributed attention:

Walk around the circle slowly when you are guiding them with your voice. don't walk constantly, pause in a place and start by walking again and pause in another place so that they know you are around them and your attention is distributed evenly among them.

6-Safe, comforting touch:

Touch them gently in their shoulders, or lift their legs gently to relax their spine and lower back, touch their head gently to give them support and comfort, push gently their hand so that their shoulders relaxes, put some imaginary magic powder making a funny noise so that they close their eyes. All these little attentions from time to time, makes them feel safe and more relaxed.

7-Suiting music:

Playing soft, gentle music is always helping along your guided voice.

Also keep these following points in mind during relaxation time:

-Make sure that you first create a suitable space & atmosphere for relaxation exercises. You better dim the lights and create a safe & warm space for kids to have enough trust to relax.

-If you are working with a new group who still don't know their yoga class well or they are not also familiar with each other, it is better to wait for a few sessions then take them into the journey of relaxation in their circle. Being unfamiliar with the surrounding space, causes tension in children. After a few sessions, when children got to know each other and the classroom better, then relaxation exercises would be more effective.

-Before starting such exercises, you may ask children to walk a bit around the classroom first, You can also suggest that they can take a favorite blanket or pillow if it makes them feel more safe and relaxed, Then ask them to lie down in any form you are inviting them due to your class theme. Your voice, the words and expressions you use are very important and you should be very mindful about how you transmit your message when you take them into a state of relaxation.

-After each relaxation exercise, it is important to ask children about their experience during the exercise. This teaches them to express their inner emotions, thus understand these emotions better. More important is that you should pay equal attention to everyone.

-All children should listen to each other's sharing, and no one should speak or judge while another one is speaking. This should come into your class agreements or rules we talked about at the beginning of this training book. Then you just refer to the rule. You can also use a magic wand, a feather, a Totem, a crystal or anything meaningful for you and your class then you can add the rule that "The one who has the chosen object can only talk, while the other listens and waits for their turns".

-If a child is restless and doesn't stay calm during relaxation, don't worry! I have some tips that might help in these situations but most of all, stay calm and just try to understand the kid and keep your positive attitude. They're always a way and patience is the key!

Now, Let's explore few solutions:

- Ask kids to do some freestyle dance, or shaking or running before you ask them to lie down. Sometimes kids have excessive energy and they need to get tired to be eager to relax. Usually when you have a dynamic class, it's easier for kids to relax at the end.

- Music always helps. You can play some fast music and ask them to shake their bodies like jellyes then play soft music and ask them to close their eyes and guide them into relaxation due to your chosen theme.
- A gentle touch as mentioned above, a positive attention can also help. But keep in mind to pay equal attention to children and don't let yourself be distracted by one child so that you put over attention to that child and ignore other kids.
- The reminder of a praise will also help, but as we mentioned you don't want to make a habit out of it, you can remind them that if they collaborate and stay in a relaxed position for demanded time in the 4 following sessions, then they will receive a surprise gift.

If the restless child keeps insisting, you can talk to him privately and ask him kindly, explaining the situation and sharing your feelings and expectations about the situation. you can also give him a secret mission, such as detecting some points of the story, or distributing the imaginary magic powder among kids...Giving him a sense of responsibility mostly works as in most cases kids who act in unexpected ways, they seek for your attention. You can make them understand that you won't pay attention to their misbehaviour but you are giving your attention first equally to all kids and you always notice and appreciate when they collaborate and do something with good intentions in class. For more about this subject you can go to the chapter we already been through together about "challenging children and how to behave?"

Using Relaxation Exercises in schools:

In today's world children face many tensions. They spend a long time in school, and despite having break time, they don't have enough time to relax. The same is for the elementary school children. After the compressed program in school, they usually try to relax at home by sitting in front of TV, Ipad, computer games...Such children often have sleeping problems.

Relaxation exercises which are presented here are also practicable in school classes. In school class, instead of lying or sitting on the ground, these exercises are done while they are sitting on desks and their feet are in contact with the ground; they put their hands either on their stomach or on their knees while their palms face the ceiling.

Experience has shown that sometimes children are too restless in the class; 5-minutes of relaxation could be more useful in calming them rather than a long speech.

1-Shake & Lose

Necessary equipment: Mats

This game teaches the children how to relax their muscles and bodies. After playing this game, they will be able to feel the peaceful effects of it on their bodies.

This practice is played in this order:

One child lies down on their back. The other child moves the first child's legs and hands to feel the resistance and the contraction of their muscles. The children learn that with the help of trusting in each other they can free their muscles and feel pleasant in their bodies.

Have them work in pairs. Sam lies down on his back and Leyla sits next to him. Sam tries to totally free and relax his body, and Leyla puts her hands on Sam's legs. At first, she doesn't pick Sam's legs up off the ground but just trembles Sam's legs with both her hands. As Sam's body is totally relaxed, his legs tremble easily. Then Leyla can pick Sam's leg up while her hands are on his calf muscles, shaking Sam's leg gently until it swings very loosely. During this exercise, Leyla should be careful that there is no extra pressure on Sam.

Leyla also shouldn't misuse Sam's trust and drop his leg suddenly or put a lot of pressure on his leg. Thus, they work on their muscles in turn and help each other to generate a peaceful and joyful feeling in their bodies.

Variation of the game

As the children become familiar with this game, they can play it in groups of three or five as well. One child lies down on the ground and the others move their legs and hands at the same time.

2-Sense of Heaviness

When the body is calm and relaxed, a sense of warmth and heaviness occurs. By concentrating on the sense of warmth and heaviness, you may help relax your body.

Encourage the children to learn the techniques so that they could use them whenever they need to relax their minds and bodies. In this exercise the children lie down on their backs, on the ground in the "resting" position.

Ask them to listen to your voice with their eyes closed. Talk very slowly and smoothly:

"Focus on your toes first, how are they feeling?"

"What do you feel in this part? Heat? Cold? A sense of tingling? Other feelings?"

"What do you feel? Do you feel heaviness in your legs? How about heat?"

"Imagine the hot sunlight is shining on your toes. Then move this imagination from your toes up to the rest of your body." Name all your body parts and guide the children to feel heat and cold in those parts.

The ankle, the shin, the knees, the thighs, hips, the belly and the belly button. When you reach to the belly, talk about breathing as well as the feeling of warmth and a sense of heaviness.

Tell them:

"Feel your belly as it goes up and down with your breaths. Just like the ocean's waves. Your belly button goes up and down slowly. Then continue the flow to the upper side of your body."

"The back, the hands, the shoulders, the neck and finally you reach the head." Never tell them to feel warm in their heads. A warm head causes headache and tension. Make them feel cool in their heads instead of heat.

"Imagine a cool breeze hitting your forehead, and feel your head heavy, and your forehead cold." After staying in this position for a while, end the exercise in this order:

"Now wiggle your fingers and your toes slowly, take a deep breath and bring your hands above your head and stretch your body from the top to the bottom."

"Then sit up slowly and explain about your experience in this sense of heaviness and relaxation."

Variation of this exercise

Follow the same structure with this exercise by transferring the feeling of lightness in your whole body.

3- Contraction & Relaxation in the Body

One of the keys to relaxation is to understand the contraction in the body.

This exercise makes it possible for children to compare the sense of contraction with relaxation. When they distinguish between contraction and relaxation in their body, it would be easier for them to relax.

Ask them to lie on the ground and first, same as we used in the Heaviness exercise, release all body parts. Then ask them to gently lift their left leg just a few centimeters from the ground, pull it forward and then release it. They can repeat it several times. Encourage them to be aware of what is happening in their muscles and respiratory system, while their legs are lifted then released. Ask them to gently lift their other leg as well and repeat the same. Then guide them as follows:

*"Be aware of the feeling in each of your legs; are they different?

Watch if one of your legs is heavier, lighter, warmer or colder than the other?

Do you feel a sense of tingling or itching in one of your legs? Do you feel one of your legs is longer than the other? heavier or lighter?

Now, guide them in the same way to contract and let go in their arms.

Then you can ask them to lift their bottom with an inhale, then release with an exhale.

Breath in, lift up the chest, then breath out, release.

You can ask them to imagine all their face muscles retract on the top of their nose! meaning to contract the whole face then let go!

bring the shoulders up to your ears then take it down and stretch your arms again by pulling it down to let go of the contraction.

After you guide them into contraction and relaxation in different body parts.

you can then invite them to come back, sit up and talk about the exercise;

4-Golden Light

Focusing on all body parts is very important in this imaginary exercise. Thinking positively creates a light, dynamic feeling in the body.

Ask the children to do this exercise while sitting or lying on the ground, and guide them in this order:

"Observe your natural breath and feel your breath becoming slow and calm. "Now pay attention to the top of your head and imagine that a Golden light is shining on this part. This light is gradually approaching your crown and entering from this point into your whole body. This white light moves all around your body, provides you with energy and power, and you find that you are stronger. First, feel the Golden light on your head, then this light slips toward the throat and after that, it reaches your chest and heart. You can feel the light in your shoulders and guide it to your palm alongside your hands. Now your palms are bright and shiny. If you feel tension or cramp in any part of your body, drag the Gold light there and imagine that the contraction is going out from your fingertips."

"Now feel the Golden light around your navel, on your belly and in all your hips and back. Continue as long as your feet are also filled with this beautiful shiny light. Now imagine that your whole body is covered with this Golden light.

You feel safe and warm, and your breathing is getting more and more slow and relaxed.

This exercise takes around five to ten minutes. After finishing the exercise let the children stay there for a few minutes. Then ask them to get out of their positions gently by moving their bodies slowly, then sit up and invite them to share their experience with the group.

5-Ball of energy

In this exercise, children learn how to transmit energy to different parts of their body through concentration. Ask the children to lie on the ground in a circle next to each other, keep their eyes closed and take the palms of their hands toward the sky. Then guide them as follows:

"Focus on your left hand and imagine that you are holding a small ball of light in your left hand. This ball provides you with light and energy and a sense of warmth flowing through this light into your body. Imagine that the light flows from the palm of your hands toward your little finger, ring finger, middle finger, forefinger and finally your thumb.

Now the light goes from your thumb to the wrist, then to forearms, arms and neck. Feel that the left hand is warm. The light is transmitted from the palm of your hand to the whole left side of your upper body, and you can feel the suiting warmth of that light in the whole left side of your upper body."

Then continue the guidance toward the right hand: "Now a small ball is on the palm of your right hand and you feel warmth and energy in this part. Like what you did on your left side, spread the pleasant warmth in each of your fingers, wrist, forearm, arm, shoulders and neck. Now place your warm and energy-filled hands on any part of your body you think needs that light to feel better and at peace."

You can continue your guidance into the flow of energy going to the legs and lower body.

In this practice, children learn to guide the required energy to the parts of the body which needs it more.

After a few minutes, ask the children to come out of this position and sit without opening their eyes. Then ask them to open their eyes gently, and share their experience with the group.

6-Colorful Bubble Of Light

Ask children to go around the room and find a safe and comfortable place to lie down. They can have their own blanket or whatever object they feel safest with. Guide them to concentrate on their breath and relax. Then guide them as follows:

"Imagine a colour making you feel safe. Now imagine a bubble of light with your chosen colour around you. You are now in this bubble, you become lighter and lighter as the bubble rises up to the sky. You are safe and protected and nobody can enter into your bubble unless you let them. Start to go explore with your bubble..."

Now, you can take them anywhere, for example, to the ocean, into space, and keep emphasizing how safe and protected they feel in their bubble. This will help them to not get scared when they imagine themselves going to all the different places using their imagination. After 5-10 minutes, slowly guide them back and out of their bubbles where they built their trust and felt safe. Then invite them to share their experience. Ask about their colours and how they felt with their chosen colour in this exercise.

You can tell them that whenever they feel they need their privacy and that they don't want others to come into their private zone, or when they feel scared or bored etc, they can use this meditation and imagine their colourful bubble around them and feel safe and protected in it.

7- The Magical jungle

Use this meditation in sessions with the theme of Jungle. Tell them that after spending a long day in the Jungle, now it's time to lie down on the ground. You can either tell them to lie on their back or maybe depending on your story ask them to go to any relaxing posture they choose or you ask them to relax.

"Imagine you are lying down in a vast green space in the middle of your magical jungle. Your body is relaxed and it's time to take a rest after a long journey full of adventures in the magical jungle. Look around; see the flowers, trees and animals. Remember the fun games you have played, laughters & joyful moments you spend in the jungle with your friends… Now this adventurous day is coming to an end and the sun is setting…."

Guide them to recall and review the events and games. Colors, games, feelings they have experienced, asanas they have learned, animals they have been playing the roles and…then continue like this:

"In the magical jungle there lives a tender-hearted angel; kind and playful. Now the angel is slowly approaching you and sparkles some of her magical dust on your palms. When you receive the magic dust, put your hands on your heart and make a wish from the bottom of your heart. Then send some of the magic to your loved ones and anywhere in the world you want to share your magic with and maybe heal someone or something who needs your magic. share your magic and the secret of this magic dust is that as much as you share it into the world you will receive more and more of the magic dust in your heart…After all you are a magical being!"

Now you can play soft music, go to the children one by one and put some imaginary magic dust on their hands. Making a sound for the dust when poured on their palms, helps them to imagine the feeling of energy in their hands, also it's really fun for them to hear the sound and always makes them smile! You can also bring some organic magic sparkles with you or shiny starts, a drop of a natural essential oil, or anything you can create or come up with the idea using your creativity. Then gradually guide them to come back, sit up and ask them to share their experience with the group.

8-Melting Ice cubes turning into a rainbow

This imaginary relaxation story helps to remove contractions; it creates a sense of freedom and lightness in the body in a colorful and joyful way.

Once kids are lie down on their back and you prepared them for the guided relaxation begin as follows:

Imagine you are a colorful ice cube!

You are solid and frozen.

First tell me:

What is your color?

Do you have a flavor? If so, what flavor are you?

How do you feel as an Ice cube!?

Now, Imagine there is a shining sun, reflecting its warm ray of lights on you, warming you & gradually you are melting and becoming now in liquid form like a colorful river. Obviously becoming a liquid you are lighter and you are flowing on the ground…As the sun keeps shining on you, You are becoming even lighter and transforming into a big, fluffy cloud going up and up, floating now in a beautiful blue sky…"""

Let them experience the sense of lightness and floating in the sky as a cloud for a while. Then continue as follows:

"Now, being the big & puffy cloud as you are, drop your colored magic sparkles from your cloud into the earth, like rain drops falling with the color of your cloud. What is your magic you are spreading into the earth now?...Love? Kindness? Happiness? Excitement? Friendship? Courage? Peace?…Now…Look at the sky! From the raindrops of all the colorful clouds a big, shiny rainbow has formed into the sky!

This rainbow is the outcome of your magic! You make the world a more beautiful place by sharing your true colors into the earth. Like this rainbow… Anyone who sees this rainbow will smile and with each smile, your world is becoming more beautiful and colorful just because of your big and generous heart."

Then, step by step guide them to come back, sit in their circle and share about their experience.

9- Magical yoga carpet

Ask the children to lie on their back on their yoga mats and get ready for the relaxation practice, guide them as follows:

"As you are lying, on your yoga mat, imagine your yoga mat is like a magical, flying carpet and it's going to take you into an adventure! Now imagine the color you want your mat to have. A color you like and feel safe with, then close your eyes. This mat is a magical mat!

What kind of magic do you receive from your mat?

Kindness?

Happiness?

Peace?

Excitement?...

You feel light and safe on this mat and this magical mat with its specific color protects you. Now slowly slowly imagine yourself flying up to the sky with your magical mat!

Where would you like to travel to?

Where would you like to share your magic power? Is there anyone specific you'd like to send your magic to? Or maybe some place on the earth which might need your magic?

Animals? plants? people? Where would you like to fly and share your magic sparks with?

As you are flying above the sky, imagine you are pouring your magic into some unhappy people and share some of your happy magic with them. I'm sure you'll bring a smile on their faces with your magic. Pour it into the oceans, the jungles & forests, to animals and other people you see from above and share your amazing healing, magical lights with your planet earth…"

Then slowly guide them back to land with their magical mats on the ground and gently ask them to move their toes and fingers then stretch their bodies, slowly coming back. Ask them about their colors and let them share about their experience. Remind them that they always have that magic power in their hearts and whenever they'll need it they can just put their hands on their heart and remember the magic. Then don't also forget to share it with others as a secret.

10-Travel to the Depths of the Ocean

This guided relaxation can be used in the session with ocean theme. However, you should note that probably some children might be afraid of water and the ocean. To create the sense of security in them, you may visualize a bubble of light or the company of a kind dolphin friend who will protect them during the inner journey into the ocean.

You can guide them into the journey on the depth of the ocean as follows:

"Lie on your back as if you are a starfish lying on the sands of the shore of an ocean. move your hands and legs as a shiny star. Now, relax your body and gently close your eyes and get ready to travel together into the depth of a beautiful ocean.

Imagine that you are lying on soft and warm sands near the ocean. Waves are slowly coming toward you. The shiny sun is caressing your skin with its warmth. You hear the sound of the waves (Here you can play music with the sound of the ocean). You also hear the sound of dolphins. Dolphins! Those nice friends that are waiting for you in the ocean.

One dolphin who is your special friend is going to take you to this amazing journey….

The waves gently pick you up and slowly take you to your friend, the dolphin, who is so excited to see you, jumping up and down on the waves and calls you with a smile. You are playing on the waves together with your dolphin friend for a while.

Now, you are getting ready to go to the depth of the ocean. If you feel safe enough just jump on the back of your dolphin friend and we're going to dive deep within the ocean. Or if you still feel a little concerned about your journey and want to feel totally safe and protected, imagine a bubble of light with your chosen color around you. No one and nothing can enter your bubble unless you give them permission. You are totally safe and protected in your bubble of light.

Now that you're ready, along with the dolphin friend start your journey to the depths of the ocean. In the depth of the ocean, there is a colorful world – Red corals, different colorful fishes, Shels, colorful herbs...and what else do you see in the depth of the ocean? Today we traveled into the ocean so remember all the creatures we played and now you visit them in your creative journey. They are all your friends and they are happy to see you...Remember that you are totally safe and protected and nothing can happen to you...Along the way you are in the search of a magical seashell. Inside the seashell, there is a surprise gift for you. This gift is like a secret! Look if you can find the shell?

Can You find it?! yes!!! Now, as you open the shell inside of it you find a shiny, colorful pearl! Especially for you! let your heart brighten from its light. Now your heart shines like a star and here is a secret nobody knows! You have a special pearl in your heart! This is the gift of the ocean to you. As you take it with you into your life, you can shine your heart secretly to the world with your gift…"

Let them remain with their magic for a while and feel it in their heart. Then gradually take them back into the shore and continue as follows:

"Now say goodbye to your friend, dolphin. If you like, you can hug your friend dolphin and know that whenever you want you can go back and meet again. you just need to close your eyes, put your hands on your heart, remember the gift of the ocean, call your dolphin friend and he'll be there for you"

Now gently guide them back to class and let them share about their experience. Ask them what kind of pearl they received and what was their mission and magic to share into the world through their gifted heart.

11-The Casket of Wishes

As You ask them to lye on their mat and relax their bodies, here goes the story:

"Imagine that your mat is transforming into a magical carpet! A magical carpet which takes you wherever you want; Just like a flying carpet!

Today your magical mat is going to take you to the Land of wishes! It's a far away enchanted land and something special is waiting for you there.

To be ready for the journey you need to be silent and so relaxed that your mat starts to fly!..

Now that you have arrived. Take a walk around this magic land. It's a beautiful and colorful land where you see magical plants, flowers and animals around it...you also see some old caskets around the enchanted land. From afar you see the glitter of a golden key! Your key opens one of these strange caskets. You must turn and try them. Your casket might be at the top of a tree! Or at the bottom of an ocean, or maybe a kind bear is keeping it for you... where is your casket hidden? When you find it, gently open it with your key. You find a bright star in it. Pick up your star and whisper your wish to the star. Now put it wherever on your body you want, for example on your heart, in your head, in your belly, in your forehead, or you can put it in your nose! on your lips! You can even eat it! Then it will shine all through you! You can also put it in your pocket...

And then get on your magical carpet and return. Your star shines on you and makes your wishes come true."

Now step by step guide them to return and share about their experience. Tell them that the shiny star is their magic power. It's their smile, their kindness, their courage and their love. The shiny star makes their magic brighten and gives it more power.

You always remind them that their magic always exists in them and encourage them with your stories to believe in themselves and their magic within.

12-Music Orchestra

You can use this fun guided relaxation for the Music orchestra theme.

Ask the children to lie down on their mat in a row next to each other. Then tell them that all together they will create a music orchestra by making a sound for each movement. It goes like this:

The first person on the line, lifts one of her legs a few centimeters off the ground and releases it by making a sound, then the other one does the same with a different sound and so on until the last person on the line. Then from the end of the line the same goes for the other leg until it reaches the first person again. Continue the fun contraction and relaxation with a sound in other body parts: hands, shoulders, hips, chest, head, face muscles, neck. All the sound follows one after another and it becomes like a funny music orchestra!

Then you can play a calming instrumental music and ask them to close their eyes and guide them as follows:

"Listen to the music playing for you. Where in your body do you feel the music? Maybe each sound and rhythm touches different parts of your body by its vibration and creates different feelings in you? How do you feel by hearing the sounds? Just listen deeply and let the music create very slow movement in your body with your closed eyes. Like the waves in the ocean or the leaves gently moving by a soft wind. Then relax again and just listen to the music with your heart. Place your hands on your heart and listen to the rhythm of your own heart. Can you hear it? boom…boom….How is the sound of your heart? Your heartbeat is the music of your heart. Listen carefully to the sound of your heart. Then say to yourself:"

"It is so good that I exist and my heart beats in its rhythm. How beautiful is the music of my heart!"

You can listen to this music and dance with it anytime you want to. All creatures have this rhythm in their heart. Anybody's heart has its own rhythm. Your heart is like the orchestra conductor of your body.

Under its guidance, all your body parts function and dance, so that you can walk, laugh and play. Listen to the sound of your heart!"

Now you can gently guide them to come back, sit in their circle and ask them to share their experiences with you and other kids.

Practice:

Now your turn to Design new guided visualization meditations. You just must close your eyes and think of a specific place where you like to be. Wonder around this place and feel your story in your heart. Then share it with the kids with lots of excitement as if you were yourself inside the phantasy land you are reciting for them.

Here, some suggested subjects for practicing your guided meditation:

On the beach, a special magical place, rainbow, travel in the land of clouds, enchanted forest, flying carpet, starry night, on the moon, in the space, becoming a fruit tree, the fairy land, magical powder, being in nature, waterfall, blanket of light, Falling hearts, luminous blanket, laughter land, land of smiles, hollow bamboos, the world of colored stones and …

Have lots of fun, get creative and enjoy the process!

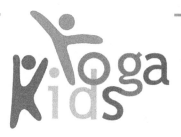

CHAPTER 18

Design Sample of a
Complete Class

At the beginning of this book you've been introduced to a time table to schedule and design your one hour and 45 minutes long sessions upon it.

Now that we covered almost the most important subjects you'll need in order to design your fun sessions, You can go through the whole sections in the book and collect the infos you need to design your yoga kids classes. Try to find as many subjects as possible and give a good thought to put your chosen teachings, games and meditations into the schedule, then time to share and practice your insights with the loving kids to whom you'll introduce a precious gift called Yoga!

Here you'll see 2 samples of a designed time table yoga kids session:

A One-hour class:

Class subject: Protecting the Environment

One of the interesting themes you can use in your sessions is Environmental Protection. You can gather information and educational activities to inform kids about the planet and how we can protect our planets by our acts. This is a great subject to consider using in your sessions. You can enhance their ecological knowledge and help them learn more about their surroundings and also boost their interest in caring for and improving the environment. They can learn and maybe reflect it also on their families.

<u>10 minutes beginning:</u>

- **Inviting children to sit in a circle**

- **Explaining about yoga**

- **Name game:** travel to cities

- **Start meditation:** A guided meditation taking kids around the globe to first explore and enjoy nature then looking at the environment, then maybe mention some obstacles the cities are facing due to environmental damages, just to inform them about the issues, like pollution, over use of plastic, overused water, energy consumption, garbage in the cities, climate change and its impact on the oceans, the forests...Whatever you mention, remember to come up with the solution during your session.

Once they understand the meaning of Environmental Protection, then you can give them the role of the Environment Protector and they will be responsible to save the planet! While they have their eyes closed, you can also give them a badge, a medallion or anything symbolic for the title of the protector to encourage their sense of responsibility.

<u>10 minutes warm up:</u>

- **Warm up game:** a walk in the city square and being guided by the traffic police (children stand in a circle. One of them will be the police and will stand in the centre with closed eyes pointing her hand forward and guide kids to go in different directions in the circle. Same as what we explored in the warm up section. you can take them along the story of going on a tour around the city and fix the problems with environmental issues. Like collecting garbage, check the car sanities, using organic products, water conservation, minimizing the use of plastic...

Below we continue with the time table and how and which games are used in the related time schedule. If you want to use this amazing theme, there are so many ideas you can come up with then add your story on it, bringing your insights into the directions and games you are giving the kids and educate them about this subject and encourage their sense of love for the nature as the fate of the planet will be in their hands, so it is actually crucial for them to be conscious about their planet and learn about how to use resources wisely to protect the planet and do their part in the battle against the climate change.

<u>25-30 min teaching asana and related games:</u>

- We can start by pointing out the rules we set. You can say like this: "Seeing the chaos we faced in our city square let's put some **rules** to give an order to the city!"

- Asana and game:

Riding a car on a subway using related games in the asana & games section, also you can use this idea: (some of the children, doing the Downward dog posture next to each other, making a tunnel under which other children pass in cat pose playing moving cars).

Going to a park nearby, using the elevator (related game in Tadasana) to reach the top of a tall tower and look at the city.

Mary-go-round game

Eating a sandwich (pastitchimuttanasa) (ex: the sandwich is wrapped in a plastic bag, we ask to not receive the plastic)

Doing different warrior postures and collecting the garbage on the ground

<u>5 minutes cool down:</u>

- Riding a bicycle to go back (cycling in the air while lying on the back position), twisting to the right and left and some leg variations like a happy baby.

<u>10 minutes relaxation and closing circle:</u>

- **Guided relaxation**: Follows with the theme remind them of their essential role in helping to have a clean and proper environment, create a vision of a clean, green, healthy and peaceful city, where all people, animals, plants and trees are happy and safe. Then congratulate them for the amazing role they had as an environmental protector.

Next, take them back in their sitting circle and have a final chat about the important subject they experienced and let them share about their thoughts and ideas on how they can protect the environment.

A 45-minute class:

- Class subject: Ocean

<u>10 minutes beginning:</u>

- Inviting children to sit in a circle

- Briefly explaining about yoga

- Talking about the ocean

- **Starting meditation**: Giving a short guided meditation with the vision of a beach and the ocean.

- **Name game:** One by one they say their name and right after they change place with another one like swimming with the waves in the ocean.

<u>5 minutes warm up:</u>

- **A fun game:** you may put some seashells and small rocks around the class and give each child a box, a sack or a basket. When hearing the music, they should go around the class, collect one shell or stone at a time put in on their mat. The rule of the game is that only one object at a time can be collected. Then when you stop the music they'll sit on their mat, count the shells and stones, put it in a side as a treasure box and tell them they can take it home with them and collect the box at the end of the class.

<u>20 minutes Asana teaching & related games:</u>

- You can first introduce the underwater creatures and ask kids to take part in naming a few, then make a shape for it in their bodies. Then show them a related posture and invite them to do the asana. To make it more fun and enhance their power of imagination, you can bring a big blue fabric and ask kids to hold the edges and make slow movements to create small waves in the ocean. Waves bring the creature on the surface and each time they will go to the related posture. The postures used in this sample class are:

Seashell (bending forward in Badakunasana or butterfly)

Shark (Shalabhasana with hooked hands in back)

Whale (Shalabhasana with open hands and legs)

Dolphin pose (Ardha Pincha Mayurasana)

Crab (Purvottanasana)Turtle (Kurmasana)

Fish (Matsiasana)

Boat (Navasana)

Group Octopus

<u>5 minutes cool down:</u>

The last creature coming out of the waves will be the Starfish! Ask kids to lie on their back with open legs and arms like a starfish. bring your hands up & down, as if the star fish is swimming to reach the sand by the ocean. Then after a few guided breaths like the angel breath we went through in the breathing section, now they lie in silence like a shiny starfish lying on the sands.

<u>5 minutes relaxation:</u>

Using the theme of ocean guided relaxation and playing a soft, relaxing music with the sound of waves and the ocean.

Practice:

Now using the instructions of the book and your own creativity, design three classes for each age group. A 45-minute class for children between 3 and 5 years of age, a 1 hour class for children between 6 and 8 years of age, and a 1-hour class for children between 9 and 11 years of age.

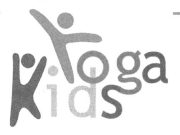

CHAPTER 19
Balancing Chakras in Children

Chakra in sanskrit language means Wheel and is pointing out to the energy centers in the body. They are like spinning colored wheels of energy. We have many of these energy centres in our subtle bodies but mainly we are influenced by the main 7 chakras positioned throughout the body, starting from the base of the spine to the crown of the head. In a healthy body the 7 chakras provide the right balance of energy to every part of the body, mind and spirit.

Balancing the chakras affect the wellbeing of our physical and emotional lives. All our habitual daily actions affect our energy body. We can balance our chakras by choosing the right diet and practices. Yoga is helping to balance these energy centres and promote a healthy body & mind.

Each chakra has its own vibration, colors and specific function in the physical and emotional body.

Here, we will briefly go through the 7 chakras; Their name, their associated color, their function then some suggested method and yoga postures also positive affirmations and sound vibrations to balance the 7 chakra in children:

First Chakra: Root chakra, named "Muladhara" in Sanskrit, is red and located at the end of the spine and is related to the sense of security and grounding and is also associated with our primal urges and also our feelings about our physical body. Dependencies, not letting go, fear of loss and anger can come from an unbalanced first chakra.

Useful practices: jumping, gentle taps on the ground with the bottom while sitting, Stamp on the ground, dancing with the sound of percussion & drum along with rhythmic breathing.

Yoga Postures: All standing postures starting with Tadasana (mountain pose). Janu sirsasana, Setubandhasana, Urdhva Dhanurasana.

Affirmation: I am strong and connected to the earth. my body is a temple for my soul. I love my body just as it is and I take care of it.

Sound: LAM

Second Chakra: Sacral chakra, "Savadhistana" in Sanskrit, is orange, located in the pelvis and is related to creativity, pleasures and sexual energy, and its unbalance results in the lack of liveliness and passion, inability, lose of appetite and in intensity can lead to anorexia. Also traumas and sudden shocks in life can block the second chakra so we can say that by balancing the second chakra we are helping to solve our unresolved emotions.

Useful practices: Making waves in the spine. Moving the pelvis. Shaking the whole body especially in the hips and pelvis area.

Yoga postures: Marjariasana (cat posture), Bhujangasana (Cobra), Trikonasana (Triangle), Ardha matsyendrasana (twist), Salabhasana (Locust)

Affirmation: I am creative.

Sound: VAM

Third Chakra: Solar plexus, "Manipoura" in Sanskrit, is yellow, located in the navel area. It is associated with the inner fire (Agni) which helps us to digest not only food but also our life experiences. Its balance results in the increase of inner power and self-confidence, a sense of happiness and its unbalance leads to lack of self worth and depression.

Useful practices: Jumping up & down like the frog posture. Push ups. Fire breaths like in lion pose and other fire breathing practices you've been introduced in the breathing chapter.

Yoga Postures: Navasana (boat), Chatuangasana Plank), Dhanurasana (Bow), Pincha Mayurasana (peacock)

Affirmation: I am confident and powerful. I can handle anything.

Sound: RAM

Fourth Chakra: Heart chakra, "Anahata" in Sanskrit, is green and located in the heart and chest area. The energies of this chakra flows into the hands and shoulders. It is associated with emotional qualities such as openness, kindness, love and forgiveness. An unbalanced heart chakra can lead to hold Grudges, loneliness, sadness and inability to give and receive love which also can provoke heart diseases.

Useful Practices: Hands on the shoulder and shoulder twist (imagination of flying like a bee), hugging oneself and moving the body (washing machine), Group hug, All the guided visualization into spreading the magic within into the world.

Yoga Postures: Matsyasana (Fish), Ustrasana (Camel), Natarajasana (Dancer), Bhujangasana (Cobra)

Affirmation: I am loved. I am love. My heart is open and I share and receive Love everyday in all possible ways.

Sound: YAM

Fifth Chakra: Throat chakra, "Vishuddha" in Sanskrit, is Blue and located in the throat, jaw, neck area. It is associated with self expression, authentic self and power of speech. If unbalanced signs will be: Hiding the true self and not giving real opinions, difficulty to express true feelings into speaking, gossiping, dominating conversations and being unable to listen to others. Also unbalanced throat chakra can result in thyroid problems and neck pain.

Useful practices: Singing, Lion breath, Jiberish talk, chanting

Yoga Postures: Simhasana (Lion), Sarvangasava (Shoulder stand), Halasana (Plough), Matsyasana (Fish)

Affirmation: I Speak my truth. I live my truth. I listen and I hear.

Sound: HAM

Sixth Chakra: Third eye, "Ajna" in Sanskrit, is purple or indigo, located in the area between the eyebrows. This chakra is related to the mind. Associated with concentration and memory, intuition, awareness in the conscious and subconscious mind, also a sense of balance in the body and mind. Since it is not yet active in small children, they cannot do easily the balancing postures. Unbalance in this chakra can lead to vision problems, lack of concentration, inability to make decisions and trust the intuition (hearing the inner voice), mental defects like ADD, ADHD, Autism, etc.

Useful Practices: Meditations, visualizations, Humming sound (Brahmi breath)

Yoga Postures: All balancing postures.

Affirmation: My thoughts are calm and peaceful. I trust my intuition.

Sound: SHAM

Seventh Chakra: Crown chakra, "Sahasrara" in Sanskrit, is white or Gold, located in the crown area. Spiritual connections get started from here, The connection with divine. When balanced one feels a sense of pure joy, gratefulness and one with the whole universe in other words connected to the source. An unbalanced seventh chakra can lead to confusion, delusion, melancholy, Brain problems and sleep disorders.

Useful practices: Visualizing a white or Gold color surrounding the crown area and expanding the light into the whole body. Massaging the head. Meditation and relaxation & yoga nidra.

Yoga Postures: Sirsasana (Head stand), savasana (relaxation)

Affirmation: I am one with the whole. The whole universe is within me. I am always safe.

Sound: AUM

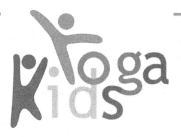

CHAPTER 20

The impact of Colors on Mind, Body and Spirit

Color is one of the languages of the Soul. We are surrounded by Colors. Any direction we look, either in a room or in a city or in nature, we see colors everywhere around us. They impact our mood and emotions. it is the colors that give meaning and life to objects and elements and make distinction between the objects in front of us. The impact of colors on our soul and mind is scientifically proved and using or avoiding certain colors is a way of self-expression. All colors have a symbolic meaning which is related to our subconscious mind and indicates how we feel inside.

Children's world is the world of colors and pure sense of rainbow emotions. Since explaining and expressing the feelings and conveying different concepts is difficult for children, we can use colors to know about their inner feelings. For example, we may ask the children: "What color do you think you are today? If you could give your feelings a color what would that color be?

There is a method of healing through colors called "Chromatherapy" or "Color therapy" in which colors are used to treat ailments. This can be through visually seeing the colors or shining the light of a related color in a particular area on the body.

Here, We're going to go briefly through some colors, their effect on our body and mind. It can help you to use the knowledge of colors first for yourself and then also in your yoga kids classes. Colors are explained in the terms of their meaning, Healing properties, Preference of colors (what does it mean when you are more drawn to this color), Aversion to color (What does it mean when you dislike or reject a color). I'll also introduce some effective crystals for each color in order for you to use the crystals if you are drawn to their energies.

*Have in mind that this is general information about the colors and is briefly described for you to be more conscious about the colors and their meanings. But there are many deeper dimensions into analyzing the colors. For example, different shades of each color can indicate a different meaning behind it, Or when you are drawn to a color or feel aversion to it, depending on your state of mind while choosing the color can hide different explanations behind it. When you are in a peaceful state of mind in your life you are usually drawn to the right color for you but when you are facing problems and the mind is disturbed you might be drawn to a color which is not advised for you to use and might increase your symptoms without you knowing it. For further analyzes and deeper insights on color therapy consult a color therapist or you can always write to me and ask your questions. I'll be happy to help you connect to your colors.

Colors and their effects:

White:

Color meaning: White is not really considered a color spectrum. The lowest hue of each color leads to white, thus white has all colors hidden in it. But in the color therapy, white has its own meaning and properties. White is a color of purification and cleansing. Also it's a color of simplicity.

Healing properties: Whenever we are lost or can not find our true colors, white can help to open the space into re connecting to our true colors within. It has a calming effect and neutralizes the energy so that the attention can be drawn in, so perfect for meditation. Helps to balance and harmonize the body & mind.

Preference of color: Connecting to the innocence. Need to cleanse and purify. A new beginning. The connection to the truth within ourselves. *Too much using the white color, like dressing in white all the time can lead to indifference and boredom.

Aversion to color: Not wanting to acknowledge the light within ourselves. Too realistic and not wanting to connect to the unknown. Hiding in the persona and not wanting to face reality.

Effective crystal: Crystal quartz/Pearl/Moonstone/Selenite/White chalcedonia

Red:

Color meaning: Warm and stimulating. Vibrant and energizing. Is the color of base chakra so also has a grounding effect.

Healing properties: Red increases the level of energy. Bring excitement and passion. For those who are inactive and sleepy, it is very appropriate but for hyperactive children may lead to intensification of excitement and anger. Red color absorbs wealth and abundance and helps the person to strengthen his position or so-called roots in the earth. Using this color increases the courage and self-acceptance. Energizes the heart and blood circulation.

Preference of color: A happy vibrant soul and is not afraid to show it. Confident in the skin and full of energy. determined. indicate also a need for personal freedom.

Aversion to color: Might be over active. Hot tempered. lack of body confidence. Can also hide fear of rejection & being judged. Also fear of sexuality might be a reason to reject Red color.

Effective crystal: Red Ruby, Red Coral.

Yellow:

Color meaning: Is an awakening and refreshing color. Color of solar plexus chakra. symbolize the sun within. warm and powerful

Healing properties: Increases learning ability and improves memory. It is anti-depression and increases self-confidence. Connecting with the power within. Since it is suitable for reducing mind shortages, it is more used in educational institutes. The person who misuses power or is hyperactive should not use this color. Generally, red, orange and yellow are not suitable for restless people and might also provoke the sense of jealousy. Using it along with purple and green, we can modify its negative effects when there is a tendency toward it.

Preference of color: Life force, vitality, happiness and joy, shows curiosity and eagerness toward learning new things. Also shows a passion for writing and reading.

Aversion to color: A person who rejects the yellow color might be someone who is emotionally disappointed and bitter. Not trusting the inner power. Lack of ambition. Tendency toward jealousy.

Effective crystal: Amber / Citrine/Yellow Sapphire.

Orange:

Color meaning: Warm, joyful & creative. Color of Sacral chakra associated with emotions and passion for life. A kind of a child-like joy, innocent and free. Color of celebration and great abundance.

Healing properties: Increases appetite and sense of pleasure. Open to creativity and joy. Relieves muscle cramps and spasms. Help to release unresolved emotions. Improves optimism and helps in depression and sadness. Balance the sexual energy.

Preference of color: Embracing creativity, Enjoying life and loves celebrations. warmth and passion. social and dynamic. Independant and dedicated.

Aversion to color: Someone who rejects the color orange might have repressed sexual feelings or other issues with sensual enjoyments in life. Can also be the opposite intense which is over sexual, sensual or too much attachment to the materialistic sides of life.

Effective crystal: Corneleon, Orange agat, Sun stone.

Blue:

Color meaning: Cooling. Color of the throat chakra. The color of truth and wisdom. Healing and calming. It is also the color of communication.

Healing properties: Is suitable for calming the mind, comfortable sleep and cooling the body in heat. It is not suitable for depressed and low-energy people and can enhance a sense of melancholy when there is a tendency toward it. Promote the power of speech and help in self expression. Reveals the truth and can help to attract peaceful connections.

Preference of color: Peaceful mind, Being helpful and caring but prefer to keep a certain distance. Loyal and faithful. Also shows patience and sincerity.

Aversion to color: Too Disciplined and judgmental. Being hard on oneself and like to keep things in a particular order. Also shows difficulty in communicating and creating relationships and intimacy.

Effective crystal: Blue Topaz, Aquamarine, Blue Sapphire, Larimar, Angelite, Blue lace Agate.

Indigo:

Color meaning: One of the colors of the third eye. A color between dark blue and purple. Like purple is a color of intuition but also communication with the higher self. It is a cool color but as it has some rays of red in it is energizing and stimulating as well.

Healing Properties: Suitable for mental problems. Relaxed the mind. Helps to focus. It's a healing color for the eyes and the ears. It helps to use intuition for guidance. Promotes deep concentration. The dark side of the color indicates arrogance. A color for great leadership and improving the power of speech.

Preference of color: Feeling focused and balanced. Feeling concentrated. Power of communication. Being confident as a guide or leader. Feeling arrogant and too confident.

Aversion to color: Not trusting the intuition and inner guide. Lack of confidence as a leader. Fear of the unknown.

Effective crystal: Lapis Lazuli, Blue Sapphire in a darker shade, Azurite, Sodalite.

Green:

Color meaning: Is the color of Nature. It's the color of heart chakra. Generosity, Openness and Trust.

Healing properties: Green is a nurturing color. Opens the heart and gives space. It is suitable for anyone who has lost their path and doesn't have a good decision-making power; Painting a small room in green can promote a sense of openness and is suitable for those suffering from claustrophobia. It opens the heart and brings a sense of trust. Stimulate inner peace. calm the nervous system. Prevent greed and jealousy. Those who are not able to say "No" should not use green color too often, or they can mix it with pink and magenta.

Preference of color: Love of nature. Interest in plants and mother nature. Kindness of the heart. Being generous, kind and caring. Love of a warm family life. Love for Children and Animals. Time for healing. Avoiding conflicts.

Aversion to color: Might indicate feeling independent and detached from relationships. Avoiding feelings. Not wanting to go to the heart. Not trusting. Can also reflect being unable to forgive.

Effective crystal: Emerald/Peridot/Green Jade/Aventurine/Malachite.

Turquoise:

Color meaning: Turquoise is a combination of Green and Blue. The color of expression from the heart. Creativity and playfulness.

Healing properties: Increases the sense of Rejuvenation and freshness; Provokes creativity & Playfulness. gives a sense of Freedom. Opens the heart and calms the mind.

Preference to color: Feeling like a dolphin! Intuitive in a playful way without seriousness. Getting in touch with creativity and doing creative work. Love to play!

Aversion to color: Feeling severe and serious. preference to security rather than risking in life.

Effective crystal: Turquoise, Aquamarine, Apatite, Chrysocolla.

Pink:

Color meaning: Pink is a color associated with the Inner child (Self-love). The energetic location in the body is above the heart chakra where the thymus gland is. It's also the color of Romance and softness.

Healing properties: Helps in emotional healings. Self love and getting in touch with the inner child. Calming and nurturing. Soften the heart and can attract loving friendships.

Preference of color: Self love and healthy inner child. Feeling loved and nurtured. feeling soft and having a kind heart. being innocent. Feeling Feminine.

Aversion to color: Lack of self love. Wounded inner child. In women or young girls might reflect not being in touch with their femininity or denying their beauty and feminine side.

Effective crystal: Rose quartz, Rhodochrosite, Pink Tourmaline, Rhodonite.

Magenta:

Color meaning: Magenta is a deep pink color. Color of Love for everything, more like a compassionate love for all. It's also the color of beauty and dance. Goddess field.

Healing properties: Connection to the divine. Connecting with our life purpose. Stimulate heart activity. Empowers feminine leadership. A great color to embrace the goddess within. Femininity. Energizing and awakening. Invitation to Dance.

Preference of color: Feeling connected to divine. Sense of beauty and lover of dance. Feeling brave, daring and a strong will power. Focused on a goal in life. passionate and in control of the emotions.

Aversion to color: May feel challenged in dealing with strong emotions. Also might show someone who wants to avoid people with strong personalities. Feeling overwhelmed.

Effective crystal: Ruby in magenta color, Garnet, Alexandrite.

Purple:

Color meaning: It's the color of the third eye. Color of intuitive creativity. Unknown and mysterious. Connection to the soul.

Healing properties: Opens the door to mystery and makes the individual closer to their spiritual inner part. The darker this color is, the more mysterious and unknown it becomes; so it can bring fear about. If the spiritual connection within us increases, we feel more attracted to this color. Purple increases the sixth sense or intuition. In meditations, it helps us be deeper and more internalized. Mixture of purple and orange is very effective on creativity. Orange is useful for increasing creativity in what we do but purple improves creativity in inspirations. In children, orange and Turquoise colors are more suitable for creativity; light purple and lilac is much more suitable for children and causes more balance and harmony.

Preference of color: Getting in touch with the spiritual part of self. Feeling intuitive. Opening the third eye. Psychic abilities. Feeling the angels. Being drawn to meditation, mysticism, spirituality and divinity. Feeling inspired.

Aversion to color: Fear of unknown and mystery. Rejecting the spiritual side of life. Might feel skeptical and doubting the existence of the soul. Resistance for the world of dreams and fantasies. Lack of inspiration.

Effective crystal: Amethyst, Ametrine, Charoite, Tanzanite, Iolite.

Black:

Color meaning: The highest spectrum of each color is black, so like white in reverse has the most intense hue of each color in it. A color of Nothingness. Shadow. Darkest mystery. Unknown.

Healing properties: This color protects the individual. When we want to protect ourselves from unwanted energies, black could be a suitable choice. Over usage of black color, blocks the energy flow. It causes depression and increases the tendency to suicide. Interest in black color is seen a lot in teenage boys & girls because they don't yet have enough trust in themselves and black color provides them with a sense of being powerful, whereas, they are weak from inside. This color absorbs the sense of mercy.

Preference of color: Can symbolize: Depression, sadness, seriousness, darkness, death also deep meditation, mystery, secrecy and nothingness or wholeness.

Aversion to color: Might fear the unknown. Not wanting to face the dark sides of self. Also shows someone who wants to get free from all limitations and blockages. The desire to break Free and throw off all the veils.

Effective crystal: Black tourmaline, Onyx, Lava, Obsidian.

The keyword of the 12 introduced colors:

-White: Clear

-Red: Energy

-Yellow: Power

-Blue: Calmness

-Indigo: Expression

-Orange: Creativity

-Turquoise: Playfulness

-Pink: Self Love

-Magenta: Universal Love

-Purple: Intuition

-Black: Mystery

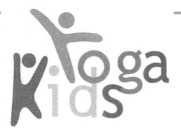

CHAPTER 21
Anatomy and Physiology for kids

It is a great idea to teach the principles of human anatomy to kids. When a child learns about her body parts and how they function She can better understand her movements. How to do that? It's super easy! First learn about your own anatomy and by taking the basic facts about bones, muscles and tissues you can turn your yoga class into an exploration of the exciting world inside a human body!

In a very simple way, what allows bones to move is the muscles contracting and relaxing.

Now, Let's learn some fun facts about the human skeleton, muscles and tissues, then use it in your designed yoga sessions for kids and make your sessions even more interesting and educative.

Skeleton

In the body of all human beings there are totally 206 bones. 8 of these bones (Cranium bones) are in the skull and their duty is to protect the brain. 14 others make the face consisting of: 3 bones in the forehead, 2 bones in the cheek, nasal bones, temporal bone, behind the ear, jaws makes it in total 22 bones in an adult human skull. In a newborn infant, there are 45 bones only in the skull which reduces to 22 in adulthood. Overall an infant has about 300 bones. Children have more bones which little by little and over time, some of these bones attach to each other and merge. This is why some of the movements children are able to make, is more challenging for adults. Also some of the baby's bones are made of a soft and flexible material called Cartilage and slowly as the child grows up the cartilage forms itself into strong bones and that's also the reason why you should not use the advanced or some of the reverse yoga postures for smaller kids. The shape of bones completes until the age of 12, but the joints are still changeable. The number of vertebrae in childhood is 33 but in adults it reduces to 26, including 24 vertebrae, 1 coccyx and 1 sacral bone. Also there are 24 ribs in the rib cage which are attached to the vertebrae. 24 vertebrae of spinal cord in order from top to bottom are as follows: 7 neck vertebrae, 12 back vertebrae, 5 lumbar vertebrae.

A child has 20 milk teeth which change into 32 permanent teeth in adulthood. From these 32 teeth, 4 of them are wisdom teeth

Scapula or the shoulder blades connect the upper arm bone with the collar bone. I like to also call it our "angel wings".

Each foot is made up of 26 bones making in total 52 bones in the feet.These bones are form 25 percent of the whole body bones.

In the hands from wrist to fingertips, there are 27 bones in each hand.

The skeletal structure of the foot and hand are similar but because the foot bears more weight, it is stronger but less movable. The bones of the foot are organized into 3 parts: Tarsal bones, Metatarsal bones and Phalanges. Similar is in the hands: Carpal bones, Metacarpal bones, Phalanges bones. In both hands and feet, each Finger and toe consists of three Phalanges, except for the thumb and big toe which have two phalanges.

Calcaneus is one of the strongest bones and tolerates 4 times the weight of the body.

3 bones named humerus, radius and ulna form hand bones. Humerus is the same arm bone which is known as funny bone. This bone connects shoulder to elbow. Radius connects elbow to thumb, and ulna connects elbow to the little finger.

The bones that make up the legs are: femore (the biggest bone of the body), patella, tibia and fibula. Femore (or the thigh bone) is a long bone extended from knee to pelvis. Tibia (or the shin bone) is extended from knee to the internal ankle and fibula, extended from knee to the external ankle. Patella or kneecap is a roughly triangular shape situated in between the shinbone and thighbone.

Some fun facts:

-The number of vertebrae of the giraffe's neck is equal to that of humans! but each vertebra of the giraffe's neck is much bigger and longer.

Nobieh Kiani fard

- The tiniest bone in the body is in the middle ear called Stapes or Stirrup.

- Femur or thigh bone is the largest bone in the human body.

-. Our teeth form part of our skeleton but are not counted bones.

-All the bones are connected to another one except one bone called Hyoid, in the throat.

In the following, the name of some of the bones of body along with the full picture of the skeleton of human body has come:

1. Skull
2. Tibia
3. Femore
4. Calcaneus
5. Clavicle/Collar bone
6. Rib cage
7. Fibula
8. Spinal cords
9. Ileum
10. Radius
11. Ulna
12. Pubic bone
13. Sternum
14. Scapula
15. Patella
16. Coccyx (tail bone)
17. Humerus
18. Phalanx
19. Sacrum
20. Pelvic floor

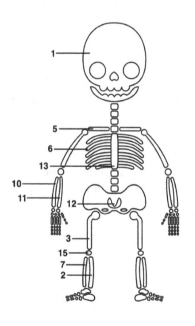
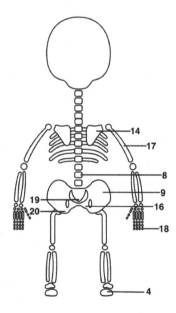

Muscles

The word muscle is derived from the Latin Musculus. Musculus in Greece or Latin means "small mouse". This name is probably chosen because of the shape of muscles. Muscles form 40 to 50 percent of the weight of the body. Thickness of muscle tissue is 15 percent more than lipid tissue.

In our whole body we have around 600 muscles.

When frowning, 43 muscles get involved and when laughing, 17 muscles. Our tongue has 8 muscles which are the strongest ones.

Muscles begin to take shape from adolescence, so before puberty, heavy body building activities should not be performed on them, because they haven't still got the shape of a complete muscle.

Muscles have a great role in our body. They are attached to the bones by connective tissues named tendons, and bones are connected to each other by the help of connective tissues named ligaments.

We have 3 types of muscles in our body: Skeleton muscles which are attached to the bones and make physical movement possible, smooth muscles which are the muscles of internal organs like the muscle of intestine, peptide and…cardiac muscles which manage the permanent movement and pumping of the heart.

It is the muscles that let us move and shape our body. If muscles are omitted, all the bones will fall on the ground. Active, conscious and strong muscles can help us with easier physical activities.

The strongest muscle of our body is the tongue, and the most laborious one is the heart which is constantly pumping blood. The bulkiest muscle is the Gluteus which is extended from the top of the thigh to the bottom of the waist. The smallest muscle like in the bones is the one in the middle ear called Stapedius. The most active muscle is the eye which moves about 100 thousand times a day and finally the tallest muscle is the one which extends from the bottom of the chest to the back of the knee and connects the leg to the body. This muscle is called psoas.

One of the muscular diseases which might occur in special children, like children with mental retardation, is "Hypotonia" or muscle loosening. To help the loosened muscle to improve, working on them without pressure could be useful.

It is worth saying that taking one step, 200 muscles of the body get involved.

Here, we introduce some of the main muscles of the body:

1. Sternoid (sternocleidomastoid)
2. Tibialis anterior (connector of tibia to the first metatarsal)
3. Quadriceps
4. Psoas (the tallest muscle of the body extended from the bottom of the chest to the back of the knee)
5. Abdominal muscles: Oblique/Rectus
6. Pectoralis major
7. Triceps
8. Deltoid
9. Latissimus dorsi
10. Diaphragm (the muscle which separates the chest cavity from the stomach cavity)
11. Gluteus marinus (maximus/medius/minimus)
12. Hamstring
13. Soleus
14. Cardiac muscle
15. Gastrocnemius (calf)
16- Trapezius

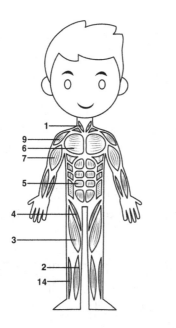
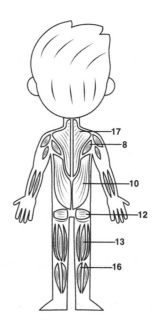

Tissues

You may know that an important part of the body is related to the tissues. Tissues are some similar cells which connect different parts of the body for a special function. Types of tissues consist: connective tissues, muscle tissues, nervous tissues and epithelial tissues (Skin). From among these tissues, connective tissue is of a specific importance. This tissue is responsible for connecting bones and muscles.

Connective tissues consist of 3 main part:

- ligament, which is responsible for connecting bones to each other

- Tendon, which connects muscles to bones

- Fascia, which is responsible for connecting muscles to each other and to blood vessels and nerves. This tissue has a very important role in connecting organs to each other.

There is another form of a tissue called Cartilage, mainly made of collagen. It's a firm tissue but it's way more softer and flexible than the bones. Cartilage is found in many areas in the body including joints in between bones in the elbows, knees, wrists and ankles. Also at the end of ribs, between vertebrae in the spine, ears and nose.

Most body tissue in children is cartilage. Children between the age 3 and 5 have very soft bones due to having a lot of cartilage tissue. Hanging poses or high stretches should be made cautiously because they might cause the joints to be overly opened and damaging to their sensitive and undeveloped bodies.

Final words

My loving friend, I really hope that you enjoyed the journey of yoga into the colorful, creative and magical world of kids with me.

How amazing it is to bring the gift of yoga to the kids who are the creators of our future on planet earth. By giving them love and support, helping them to know their body and mind through yoga you are touching their soul and heart. You might not change their whole life but in these few moments of delightful yoga sessions, you can affect some part of their collective consciousness and touch their souls in a way that might change their whole destiny leading them to growing up into more conscious adults. As our sweet friend Winnie the Pooh said:

"Sometimes, said Pooh, the smallest things take up the biggest room in your heart" Winnie the Pooh.

The whole life is a play, a "leela" which means God's play through us. Let your heart guide you. Go back to your innocence. Embrace your inner child and let it lead your life. Live your true essence and then only share your magic sparks with the kids who will see the world through you. Let them see the magnificence of a life guided by conscious, loving, playful, compassionate souls.

Enjoy the fun and magical moments you will spend working with children. You will cherish them your whole life and the magic sparks will shine through you and all the kids who take the ride along with you.

Wish you an amazing experience and hope to hear from you soon.

Nobieh Kiani fard

Let me know how your experience was on applying the insights from this book into your own personal life and your insights on working with kids. I'll be enchanted to hear from you!

With love & plenty of colorful magic sparkles!!!

Om Shanti,

Nobieh
www.nobiehkiani.com

Acknowledgment

First of all, I want to thank all my beautiful teachers and students during all these past 20 years for the delightful moments we shared together. All your love and support helped me to sing my heart songs into the world!

And a special thanks to "Hedieh Kianyfard", for all her unconditional Love and support. My most beloved sister who is the greatest, precious Gift of my life as her name reflects her true essence which means "Gift". Love You with all my heart! None of the magic would be possible without you...

Thank you!

References

1. *Yoga for children: A complete illustrated guide to yoga by Swati Chanchani*

2. *How to talk so kids can learn 1, 2, 3 by Adele Faber & Elaine Mazlish*

3. *Recovery of your inner child by Lucia Capacchione*

4. *The new child by Osho*

5. *Yoga games for children by Danielle Bersma & Marjoke Vissche*

6. *Yoga kids by Marsha Weing*

7. *Yoga for children by Mary Stewart*

8. *Once upon a pose by donna freeman*

9. *The ABC's of Yoga for kids by Teresa Power*

10. *Improve games for children & adults by Bob Bedore*

11. *Movement games for children: Fun and learning with playful movement by Huberta Wiertsema*

12. *Yoga adventure for children by Helen Purperhart*

13. *Yoga for the special child by Sonia Sumar*

14. *Partner yoga by Cain Carrol*

15. *Shel Silverstein*

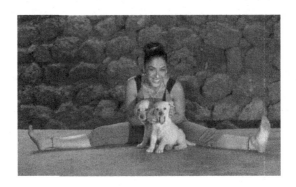

Author's Biography

Nobieh is an international yoga and dance instructor and Workshop Organizer. Owner of NOBIEH school of yoga registered with Yoga Alliance since 2014. Founder of a conscious dance system called "Dance Of No Name", author of the book by the same title "Dance Of No Name".

She is also an Independent Natural Artisan Perfumer.

She has taught yoga for two decades, travels internationally training kids and teachers on advanced yoga. She also carries out yoga and dance workshops, and training to group therapies. In doing all of these, she sells her natural perfumes and jewelry collection around the world.

Her starting point with yoga was IYENGAR style…For a couple of years she was assisting, then teaching with a Senior Iyengar yoga teacher in her home country, Iran.

Then she started to teach yoga to children and as she is saying it herself:

"I am always so grateful for the gift of sharing my passion at the beginning of my journey to kids, as they taught me the real meaning of meditation which is to be totally present in That moment…"

Those early experiences of teaching yoga to children took her into journeys of learning more about the psychology of connecting with kids, color therapy, getting more and more creative in the process of her learnings, diving more into inner child therapy works &… Also like everything else in her own life, she sees abundance as well in Yoga…So she never limited her teachings into just one style of yoga and she explored different styles, methods to connect with her nature which is creative, dynamic, intuitive, fun, colorful, modern with lots of respect to keep the real aspects of the traditions in which she was learning about…

All those experiences lead her to create her own Yoga kids TTC (Teacher's Training Course) which today she offers in Nobieh school of yoga registered with yoga alliance since 2014.

"It's been an honor to educate teachers globally and witness how they get in touch with their own inner child, mostly as they refer to this program "A life changing experience"...Also bring the joy of yoga into other children in their own time and unique creative way…"

Nobieh

www.nobiehkiani.com